Contents

Towards a healthy district

Organizing and managing district health systems based on primary health care

E. Tarimo

Director, Division of Strengthening of Health Services,
World Health Organization, Geneva, Switzerland

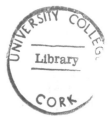
World Health Organization
Geneva
1991

WHO Library Cataloguing in Publication Data

Tarimo, Eleuther
  Towards a healthy district : organizing and managing district health systems based
  on primary health care.

  1. Community health services – organization & administration
  2. Health planning 3. Primary health care – organization & administration I. Title

ISBN 92 4 154412 0   (NLM Classification: WA 546.1)

TYPESET IN INDIA
PRINTED IN ENGLAND
89/8299—Macmillans/Clays – 5500

Preface

In many parts of the world, progress towards the goal of health for all by the year 2000 is slow and uncertain. While most countries have formulated broad policies, strategies and plans for achieving the goal, the implementation of these plans is often weak. The current efforts of numerous agencies and sectors to extend health care will succeed only if each district can identify its own priorities and target the available resources to the individuals, families, communities, and other population groups who are underserved or at risk. The need to adopt a population approach and to identify the target groups for health programmes is the point of departure of the present publication.

The ideas presented here are based on a number of years' experience as a district health manager, as well as on extensive discussions and consultations with colleagues both within and outside WHO. I am particularly grateful to Dr G. Fowkes, Department of Community Medicine, University of Edinburgh, Edinburgh, Scotland, and Dr Asamoah Baah, Ministry of Health, Accra, Ghana, for their helpful suggestions, as well as to the many individuals who commented on the early drafts of this book.

E. Tarimo

Introduction

In May 1977, the Member States of the World Health Organization adopted the goal of "Health for all by the year 2000". If this goal is to be achieved, the people who do not currently have access to appropriate health care—those still missing from the "all" in "health for all"—must be identified, and services must be developed to meet their needs. The most practical unit for doing this is the district, where—given coordination by means of good planning and management—health professionals, auxiliaries, workers from other sectors, and community members can assume collective responsibility for the health of the community. Unfortunately, this team potential is seldom realized. District plans are often poorly formulated or non-existent, targets are vague, and efficiency, effectiveness, and quality of services are seldom considered. The activities of various programmes and institutions continue to be piecemeal and poorly coordinated, while health services are concentrated in particular areas, leaving large population groups with little or no access to health care.

This publication is concerned primarily with orienting health care workers in district health systems in developing countries to ways and means of overcoming problems, and describes briefly how district health systems can be improved. It is not meant to be a comprehensive or detailed manual, but rather a stimulus to action and to the acquisition of skills for the improvement of district health systems.

It is addressed primarily to those directly concerned with improving health within a defined population, and particularly to members of district health management teams. It should also be relevant to provincial, national, and international institutions concerned with the role of primary health care in improving health. In examining the organization and management of district health systems, the book focuses on nine issues, each of which is an integral part of a district planning cycle (Fig. 1), and which address the following sets of questions:

- Does the country have national policies, strategies and plans of action for health for all? Are support and guidance provided to districts?

1

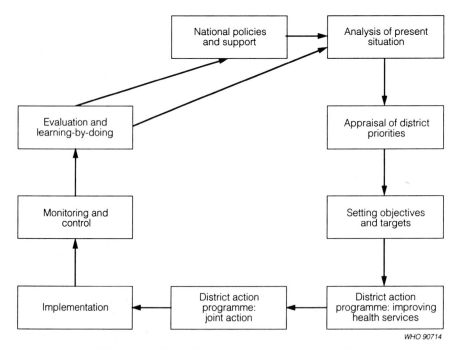

Fig. 1. The district planning cycle

- Are basic data on the characteristics of the population, level of health, major health problems and coverage with essential health care readily available in the district?

- Have district priorities been appraised?

- Have objectives and targets for health and health care been set?

- Does the district have an action plan for important programmes such as health promotion, maternal and child health, school health, environmental sanitation, occupational health, control of diseases and curative services?

- Are there effective mechanisms to get everyone — communities, health-related sectors, nongovernmental organizations and the various health programmes — to work together?

- Are there adequate resources, incentives, logistics and organizational arrangements to ensure prompt implementation of programmes?

- Are activities monitored and controlled regularly? Is there a mechanism for quality assurance?

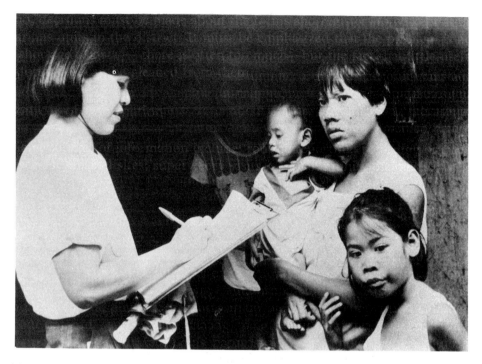

A health worker in the Philippines adds another piece to the jigsaw of a nation's health. *Photo WHO/Zafar (19938)*

- Is periodic evaluation carried out? Are efforts made to find solutions to problems encountered?

If the answer to most of these questions is "yes" for a given district, it is already well on the way towards becoming a healthy district. If not, this book provides suggestions and pointers as to what could be done to improve the situation.

Some definitions

What is a district?

The district is the most peripheral fully organized unit of local government and administration. It differs greatly from country to country in size and degree of autonomy, and population may vary from less than 50 000 to over 300 000.

It is geographically compact and every part of it can normally be reached within a day. As a unit, it is small enough for the staff to understand the major problems and constraints of socioeconomic and health development, and for health and other workers to know each other and be more humane in their approach. It is also a large enough unit for the development of the technical and managerial skills essential for planning and management. There is usually a central administrative point where the main government sectors are represented. The district is often the natural meeting-point for "bottom-up" planning and organization and "top-down" planning and support and is, therefore, a place where community needs and national priorities can be reconciled.

The district offers great opportunities for effective intersectoral action, since it is an area within which bodies such as development committees and district councils can very easily plan and act in unison. At district level, away from rigid central divisions and bureaucracies, different sectors have always tended to work together and people find it easy to collaborate on specific issues. The constitutional, legal, political, and administrative structures will determine the degree to which responsibilities will be decentralized. These structures also influence the amount of community participation through, for example, representative assemblies or other established mechanisms for the involvement of citizens in public matters.

What is a health system?

"A health system is the complex of interrelated elements that contribute to health in homes, educational institutions, workplaces, public places and communities, as well as in the physical and psychosocial environment and the health and related sectors" (*1*).

What is a district health system?

A district health system based on primary health care is a more or less self-contained segment of the national health system. It comprises first and foremost "a well-defined population living within a clearly delineated administrative and geographical area. It includes all the relevant health care activities in the area, whether governmental or otherwise. It therefore consists of a large variety of interrelated elements that contribute to health in homes, schools, workplaces, communities, the health sector, and related social and economic sectors. It includes self-care and all health care personnel and facilities, whether governmental or nongovernmental, up to and including the hospital at the first referral level, and the appropriate support services, such as laboratory, diagnostic, and logistic support. It will be most effective if coordinated by an appropriately trained health officer working to ensure as comprehensive a range as possible of promotive, preventive, curative, and rehabilitative health activities (*2*).

The network of manpower and facilities providing health care at district level varies greatly from country to country. At the most peripheral level of contact between the community and the organized health service, there are health units bearing different names in different countries: dispensary, clinic, health post, health centre, health subcentre, general practitioner's office, etc. Somewhere in the district, usually in the main town, there is a district hospital. There may also be other hospitals, often belonging to nongovernmental organizations, such as missions and societies. Within the community itself, there may be community health workers. Also, many individuals, families, groupings within communities, and other sectors will be involved in health care activities.

What is primary health care?

The expression "primary health care" has traditionally been used to mean the first-level contact between patients or communities and organized health care. In this sense, it includes the services provided by peripheral health workers, including general practitioners, nurses, and health auxiliaries. The International Conference on Primary Health Care, held at Alma-Ata in 1978, used the expression to convey two other meanings: essential health care consisting of at least eight elements (see Fig. 2), and an approach to the provision of health care that is characterized by equity, intersectoral action, and community participation. It is essentially to these two last meanings that the expression now commonly refers.

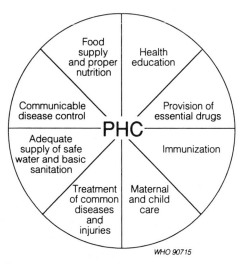

WHO 90715

Fig. 2. The eight elements of primary health care (PHC)

CHAPTER 1

National policies and support

There remain many decisions to be taken and activities to be carried out by governments to bring about necessary changes in district health care. Inequities in health and health care still prevail in many parts of the world. In spite of being committed to the goal of health for all, some countries have not as yet defined the relevant policies and plans of action, while others have produced quite inadequate ones. National plans of action must institute a fair distribution of resources and programmes throughout the country, with preferential allocation to underserved districts. They should also provide a framework for districts so that their action programmes meet their needs.

The objectives of primary health care can only be achieved if each sector makes an appropriate contribution. For this to happen effectively, a mechanism for intersectoral coordination and cooperation must be established, and this is where the central government comes in. The minister of health could, for instance, prepare a document for the cabinet suggesting possible ways and means of ensuring the desired coordination. These might include, at central level, a subcommittee of the cabinet and, at district level, a subcommittee of the district development committee. Legislation may be required to set up such mechanisms at government level.

The existence in the ministry of health of a high-level committee or focal point for the support of primary health care can bring about more general support, and an increasing number of countries are developing high-level coordinating networks to support the implementation of primary health care. These have different names in different countries, for example, national primary health care implementation committee, national health council, etc. These networks bring together representatives of nongovernmental organizations, professional associations, and technical institutions. Collaborative networks involving technical institutes, such as universities, social science institutes, and management and administration centres, might be set up for the same purpose.

In countries where the administrative system has been decentralized to district level, the development of district health systems is greatly facilitated. Elsewhere, progressive decentralization should be targeted—so many districts by 1992, so many by 1993, etc.

Financial delegation to the district is the key factor in providing opportunities for change to be initiated within the district according to local circumstances. Decentralization without delegation of appropriate financial decisions does not work. There is also a need to ensure political commitment inside districts to fiscally and socially responsible management.

Decentralization requires, first, better trained health managers at district level, secondly, a health team approach, and thirdly, planning support from the central authority in the form of guidelines and advisory staff.

Political commitment will have to be buttressed by economic support. Government expenditure on health programmes in many developing countries seldom exceeds 2% of the gross national product. The small sum spent per capita is an important contributory factor in the poor coverage of public health services. Efforts will have to be made to gain the backing of economic planners at both central and district levels. To this effect, it will be necessary to prepare a properly costed financial master-plan. Where further increases are not possible, alternative ways of financing district health systems, including cost-sharing, have to be considered.

In order to improve district health systems, a managerial process will have to be established and used at both central and district levels. In the districts, this process should be sensitive and responsive to epidemiological patterns in the community, as well as to local cultural habits pertaining to health.

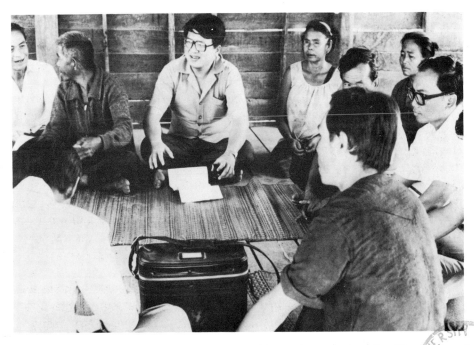

The medical officer in charge of provincial health services meets with village elders in Thailand. *Photo WHO/A. S. Kochar* (18549)

What type of support can the district management team expect from the national level?

The ministry of health should produce guidelines or protocols on district health systems which define national policies and provide planning norms for adaptation by health teams. Specific support should be offered by the central level in the following areas.

Planning and management

Central authorities can:

- set out clearly how national health objectives and health service targets may be translated into district objectives and targets and vice versa, thus helping district staff to set their own objectives more easily;

- identify the priority areas to which extra resources should be allocated, thus assisting the district staff in their own determination of priorities;

- provide experts in demography, epidemiology, etc. on a short-term basis to assist district staff in analysing and setting priorities until they have gained the numerical and other skills required to conduct a situational analysis (such expertise should be provided only until local staff are proficient in the relevant tasks);

- initiate training programmes in planning at district level, for example, short courses held at a national centre or locally, or in-service training while district staff are in the process of planning future activities (the aim should be to enable staff to make competent district plans without the assistance of outside experts);

- provide extra resources for these initiatives, or attempt to obtain them, on behalf of districts, from nongovernmental and other sources;

- provide examples of simple indicators and methods of recording, aggregating and analysing data to obtain useful information;

- provide guidelines on budgeting, cost analysis, and cost control;

- provide guidelines on technical issues, including appropriate ways of controlling important diseases.

Joint action

In addition to forming national coordinating committees, central authorities can encourage community participation, intersectoral collaboration, and the integration of vertical programmes in districts by:

- organizing more joint action at the national level, because this often leads to similar joint ventures lower down the system;

- providing earmarked resources at district level to encourage joint action;

- attempting to change the attitudes of health service staff and the general public regarding primary health care—for example through the mass media.

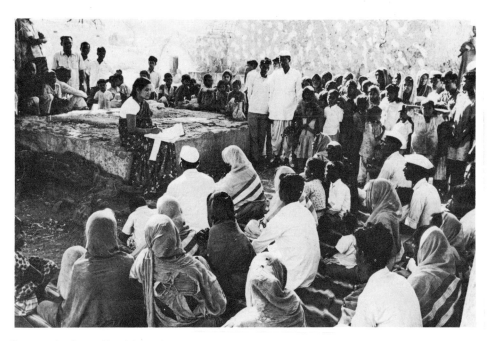

Community-based health workers are part of the primary health care strategy. Good health is not something that can be imposed from the outside. In this Indian village the entire community has gathered to discuss attitudes and appropriate action. *Photo WHO/UN (19135)*

CHAPTER 2

Analysis of the present situation

District planning is crucial if primary health care is to be improved. Because the population and geographical area of a district are of a manageable size, the information needed for planning will be relatively easy to obtain. In addition, communication and change will be easier because staff within the district will often know one another personally.

For an analysis of the present situation in the district, data on the following are required: population; health indicators; deployment of resources; and coverage. This information, which is the basis for appraising district priorities, setting programme objectives and targets, and specifying the measures to be taken, should provide an insight into overall health needs and make it possible to ascertain the strengths and weaknesses of the existing district health system and how it can be improved. Data can be gathered from routine information collected by health workers in their day-to-day work, reports of studies previously carried out in the area, and census data. Local data rather than national statistics should be used as much as possible. Incomplete data should not be discarded since they may prove useful if "enriched" and carefully interpreted. Special surveys may provide more accurate information (for example, on disease incidence and prevalence), but they are expensive and time-consuming. They should be resorted to only where better estimates are likely to lead to a change in policies and plans.

The district health team should assess in some detail the major health problems in the district and the extent to which care programmes are overcoming them. Both "strong" and "deprived" areas of the district should be identified.

Population

Where do the people live? Is this likely to affect health care coverage and utilization? How big are various population groups, i.e., the under-fives, children aged 5–14, women of childbearing age (15–44 years)? Table 1 shows how such information can be summarized.

Variations in population size between subdistricts will show what areas may need additional health facilities. The age structure of the population will help in determining the types of service required. The extent of urbanization

Table 1. Presentation of information on a district's population, by subdistrict and age group [a]

	19.. (five years ago)		19.. (current year)		Projections for 19.. (in 5 years' time)	
	No.	%	No.	%	No.	%
Total	86 000		100 000		111 000	
Subdistrict						
A	34 000	40	42 000	42	52 000	47
B	21 800	25	21 500	21.5	21 000	19
C	30 200	35	36 500	36.5	38 000	34
Urban	17 200	20	24 000	24	31 000	28
Rural	68 800	80	76 000	76	80 000	72
Age						
0–11 months	3 000	3.5	3 600	3.6	4 000	3.6
1–4 years	12 500	14.5	14 400	14.4	16 000	14.4
5–14 years	23 000	27	27 000	27	30 000	27
15–49 years (females)	19 000	22	22 000	22	24 500	22

[a] The figures given are for purposes of illustration only.

will indicate whether there is a need to develop urban-oriented primary health care (3).

Data on socioeconomic factors such as income, occupation, and educational level, which have a strong bearing on health status and health service utilization, should also be included.

Information on the following should be obtained for selected years: crude birth rate (CBR), expected annual number of births (CBR × total population), crude death rate, and population growth rate. Further parameters are given in Table 2.

Health indicators

The types of data listed in Table 2 can provide important information for comparative purposes, but are frequently not available at the district level. It is useful, therefore, to obtain approximate figures or, at least, to discover whether rates are higher or lower than the national averages. At the local level, there are usually sources of data that can be consulted, e.g., morbidity data can be obtained from hospital or health centre registers. The infant mortality rate (number of deaths of children under one year of age per 1000

Table 2. Presentation of information on selected health parameters[a]

	19.. (5 years ago)	19.. (current year)	Projections for 19.. (in 5 years' time)
Crude birth rate (CBR) (per 1000 population)	47	46	45
Expected number of births (CBR × total population)	4 000	4 600	5 000
Crude death rate (per 1000 population)	19	18	16
Population growth rate	3%	3%	3.1%
Infant (<1 yr) mortality rate (per 1000 live births)	130	120	110
Child (1–4 yrs) mortality rate (per 1000 children aged 1–4)	22	19	16
Maternal mortality rate (per 100 000 deliveries)	700	650	600
Percentage of newborn infants whose weight is below 2500 g	15%	15%	14%
Percentage of children whose weight for age is below normal	25%	24%	23%

[a] The figures given are for purposes of illustration only.

live births) is an important indicator. It reflects not only the prevalence of diseases immediately responsible for death, such as malaria, pneumonia, and diarrhoea, but also the general level of the maternal and child health services, the health of mothers, literacy, environmental sanitation, and the degree of socioeconomic development. Data should be analysed to determine the most frequent causes of death and ill-health, and trends over the previous five years. Are trends in the district different from national trends?

In addition to indices of mortality and morbidity, information may be obtained on the prevalence of certain risk factors for disease. For example, what proportion of the population obtains water from a clean supply? How many women do not breast-feed their infants? How many children are not fully immunized? What proportion of the population is malnourished or does not have access to adequate food? What proportion of the population lives near rivers and is at risk from onchocerciasis? How many people use schistosome-infested lakes? What proportion of the population smokes cigarettes or abuses alcohol? An assessment of the prevalence of risk factors in the community is important for deciding on preventive measures.

Deployment of resources

Is the number of health facilities in the district sufficient to allow for the satisfactory implementation of primary care activities? Data on the population having access to facilities within the district can be presented in tabular form as in Table 3, or by means of maps as in Fig. 3. The percentage of the population living within, say, one hour's walk or travel should be worked out for each facility. This information will point to the areas that should be given priority as regards new facilities.

Table 3. Distribution of facilities by type: tabular presentation[a]

Subdistrict population	Number of health facilities				Population per health centre/ subcentre
	hospital	health centre	subcentre	community health worker	
A 34 000	1	4	2	7	5 667
B 21 800	0	3	0	4	7 267
C 30 200	0	1	1	6	15 100

[a] The figures given are for purposes of illustration only.

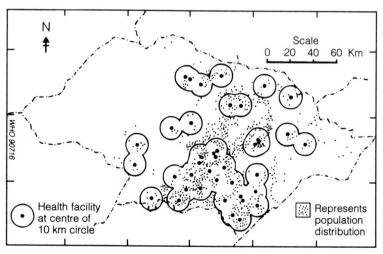

Fig. 3. Example of distribution, by district and subdistrict, of health facilities providing services within a radius of 10 km

What is the pattern of utilization of services? Are there separate units and staff for the different elements of primary health care? Do the hospitals, health centres, and other facilities have a defined geographical area of responsibility? What is their outreach to communities? What proportion of households is covered by community health workers through outreach activities? An assessment of these aspects will indicate deficiencies in the organization of services and possible corrective action.

Are there intersectoral coordinating bodies at district and village level? How effective are they? What mechanisms exist to facilitate community participation? Information on these subjects will make it possible to decide how existing mechanisms can be strengthened and whether new ones are needed.

Is the number of health personnel sufficient to provide adequate coverage of the population? What are the national norms? What percentage of established posts are filled? What is their distribution/concentration within the district by type? Are there too many of one category and not enough of others? If there are community health workers, what are their roles? Does the level of district staff approach national staffing targets? Do the staff have job descriptions? What training and in-service orientation programmes are provided? Are these adequate? Are there appropriate supervisory arrangements? Is staff morale high? If there is a shortage of drugs, which drugs are affected and what are the underlying reasons? Assessment of these aspects will indicate deficiencies in the organization of services and stimulate corrective action.

Finances

The distribution of finances within the district needs to be determined and alternative ways found of using available finances equitably. Data are often deficient and an *ad hoc* survey may be necessary. Is the per capita health expenditure in the district comparable with national per capita health expenditure? Is there a fee-for-service or other form of cost-recovery scheme in the district? How much money was generated in this way during the last fiscal year? What support is provided by outside agencies? How have funds been allocated within the district between capital (investment) and recurrent (operating) items, between facilities, and for manpower? To what extent have allocated funds been used in terms of both recurrent and capital expenditure? (See Table 4.)

Table 4. Presentation of district health budget, 1986–1990

	1986	1987	1988	1989	1990	1986–90 (% change)
Recurrent allocation (a)						
Recurrent expenditure (b)						
b/a (%)						Not appl.
Capital allocation (c)						
Capital expenditure (d)						
d/c (%)						Not appl.

The following information should also be obtained:

- Estimated financial support (separate capital and recurrent items) from other sources such as nongovernmental organizations, private enterprise, and parastatal organizations.

- Cost by facility (i.e., recurrent costs for salaries, drugs, etc.).

- Cost per contact (i.e., average cost for each outpatient attendance or inpatient stay).

- Proportion of recurrent budget allocated to hospitals compared with other services.

Coverage

Coverage is a measure of the extent to which a population entitled to a particular service, such as antenatal care or immunization, actually gets it. Coverage data should be obtained for each health facility in the subdistricts, for maternal and child health, water supply, environmental sanitation, and other services having a bearing on health. The following are examples of indicators that could be used:

- Percentage of mothers attending at least one consultation with trained health personnel during the antenatal period.

- Percentage of mothers attended at childbirth by trained personnel.

- Percentage of mothers assessed for risk factors.

● Percentage of eligible children immunized against diphtheria, tetanus, pertussis, measles, poliomyelitis, and tuberculosis.

● Percentage of children subject to regular growth monitoring.

● Percentage of population having safe water within 15 minutes' walking distance.

● Percentage of population with sanitary facilities in the house or its immediate neighbourhood.

● Percentage of population that is literate, with separate data for males and for females.

● Percentage of population having a certain minimum number of contacts with services and/or community health workers per year (e.g., two per person per year). In addition, data should be prepared on degrees of contact with health services by specific sections of the population, e.g., according to age, sex, income, and occupation.

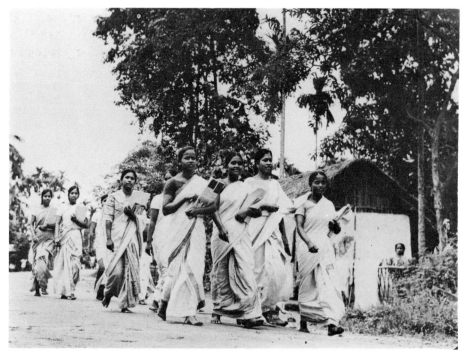

Young health professionals on the march in Delhi. One of the measures taken to improve the lot of the urban poor is to ensure that every medical student works for a time in a health centre on the fringe of the capital. *Photo WHO/N. Vohra (19120)*

The goal of coverage analysis is to identify population groups or geographical areas that are underserved, with a view to introducing appropriate remedial measures. Coverage data are most useful when presented by subdistrict and by recognizable population groups. Analysis of such data, in conjunction with data on finance, deployment of resources, health indicators, and population, can help pinpoint what changes have to be introduced in these areas in order to meet the health needs of the district. For example, if a subdistrict has a comparatively high infant mortality rate, and an insufficient number of antenatal care and other services, a redeployment of resources in favour of such services should be planned.

Urban primary health care

While primary health care applies the same principles in both rural and urban populations, the urban situation has certain special features, including rapid population increase, a high concentration but limited accessibility of health facilities and services, and the diversity of urban communities. In these circumstances it is essential to use the available resources efficiently and equitably by concentrating on disease prevention and the elimination of environmental health problems. Health education and promotion should be stressed. This calls for innovative ways of identifying and reaching groups at risk in slums and periurban areas.

CHAPTER 3

Appraisal of district priorities

Resources for health care being invariably limited, choices have to be made as to the diseases, population groups, geographical areas, and programmes that require attention. Priorities may be chosen for various political, social, economic, and health reasons. One must not delude oneself into thinking that the choice can be based solely on valid scientific evidence and that there are "right" and "wrong" decisions. Priorities will vary locally and must be based on reasonable consensus, ideally with the participation of community leaders. Fig. 4 depicts the health systems "cube". It is obvious that each of the four "dimensions" —functional infrastructure, community involvement and intersectoral collaboration, level of service delivery, and primary health care elements—can be used as a framework for setting priorities. In the case of

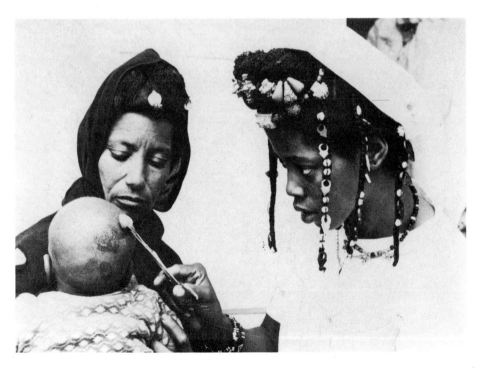

A baby is treated by a health worker at the Nouakchott Women's Union, a nongovernmental organization providing maternal and child health care in Mauritania. *Photo WHO/UNESCO/ P. Almasy (19534)*

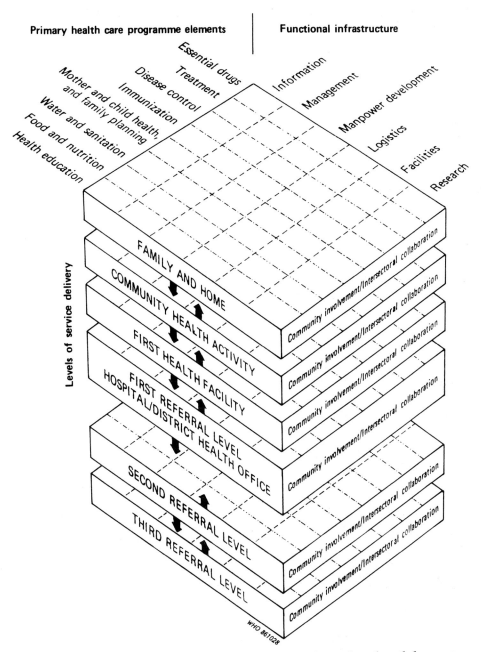

Fig. 4. A conceptual model of a comprehensive health system based on the principles of primary health care

levels of service delivery, for example, a decision must be made as to which level—home, community, local facility, or referral centre—will receive most resources.

For tackling practically any health problem and carrying out any programme, it is necessary to have a basic infrastructure of health manpower, facilities, an information system, logistic support, and continuous contact between the organized services and the community. Priority should therefore be given to strengthening the functional infrastructure. As regards population groups, the aim should be to give priority attention to those found to be at special risk.

Various techniques, such as scoring systems, should be viewed simply as methods of organizing the process of choosing priorities so that all the appropriate issues (such as costs) are considered. But adding together weights for different parameters (e.g., costs and effectiveness) is not always a good way of reaching a final decision. The chart below (Table 5) can be used to organize the choice of health priorities, with each parameter scored

Table 5. Sample priority chart[a]

Health problem or risk factor	Frequency	Mortality	Morbidity	Intervention		Priority ranking
				cost	effectiveness	

[a] Each parameter can be scored as follows:	+	++	+++
frequency in population	uncommon	common	very common
mortality (years of life lost)	low	moderate	high
morbidity (years of reduced health)	low	moderate	high
costs	very expensive	moderately expensive	inexpensive
effectiveness	ineffective	moderately effective	very effective

20

simply as +, + +, or + + + and the scores used as a guide in establishing an order of priority for specific problems.

Rather than aim programmes at single diseases, it is advisable to base priorities on risk factors or disease agents, since action to deal with these can produce a variety of benefits. For example, nutrition programmes may reduce not only the incidence of kwashiorkor, marasmus, and other diseases directly attributable to poor nutrition, but also the mortality and morbidity associated with infectious diseases. Assessing the cost-benefit of such programmes is, however, not easy, precisely because of the variety of benefits that might ensue.

Targeting the elements of primary health care

The Declaration of Alma-Ata defined primary health care as consisting of at least eight elements (see Fig. 2, p. 5). Many questions have been raised about these elements, deemed by some insufficient and by others too numerous.

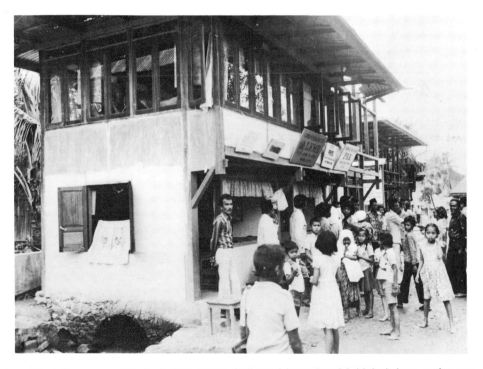

In a West Sumatran village, a little house indicated by painted initials brings under one roof a whole series of health care programmes carried out at village level. *Photo WHO/ UNICEF/M. Black (18905).*

The latter would prefer to concentrate on just two or three elements that appear particularly "ripe" for concerted action because of the availability of appropriate low-cost technology and because interventions in the areas concerned are likely to have a considerable impact on health.

In practice, the eight elements constitute a set of tasks, none of which should be neglected. The aim at district level should be to carry out essential activities in respect of each of the eight elements, within the constraints of available resources, rather than providing greater support for programmes dealing with only one or a few elements. The details (depth and content) of this task will vary from country to country. Cancer and cardiovascular diseases, for example, are very prevalent in the developed countries and considered of great importance, so that considerable resources go into providing sophisticated curative care for those who suffer from them. The developing countries, however, cannot afford to provide a similar type of care, but primary prevention of these diseases by promoting healthy behaviour—physical exercise and abstinence from smoking, for example—is feasible in all countries.

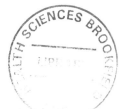

CHAPTER 4

Setting objectives and targets

Once priorities have been formulated, the next step is to specify goals. However, these goals may need frequent revision during planning and programme implementation, particularly because of the constraints imposed by lack of resources. In theory, one should start setting objectives by specifying the degree of improvement desired in respect of each health problem and then determining the appropriate level of service coverage (the operational target) needed in order to achieve it. In practice, however, it is not possible to set a realistic health objective for a given disease without at the same time considering all the other health priorities. Priority health problems should therefore be grouped together, from the service standpoint, to facilitate the setting of objectives and targets (e.g., all diseases preventable by vaccination could be considered as one group, as could all antenatal health problems) (4).

Goals can be expressed as health improvement objectives, operational targets, and health infrastructure targets.

Health improvement objectives should indicate:

– the health problem or risk factor to be addressed;

– specified changes in the health problem or risk factor;

– target dates;

– the target population.

Here are some examples of health improvement objectives:

● A specified reduction in infant mortality rate and maternal mortality rate by . . . . . (specify date).

● A specified reduction in morbidity rates from endemic diseases such as measles and malaria by . . . . . (specify date).

● A specified reduction in malnutrition rates in the under-fives by . . . . . (specify date).

- A specified reduction in disparity in health status in different parts of the district by . . . . . (specify date).

- A specified reduction in percentage of children of a specified age with dental caries by . . . . . (specify date).

- A specified increase in percentage of population with a healthy life-style, e.g., practising breast-feeding, abstaining from smoking, etc. by . . . . . (specify date).

Operational targets should indicate:

– the intervention needed for the achievement of one or more health improvement objectives;

– target dates;

– the geographical location;

– the target population.

Here are some examples of operational targets:

- Increase of . . .% in number of people knowing what constitutes a healthy life-style, e.g., proper diet, breast-feeding, cleanliness, use of latrines, abstinence from smoking, moderation in use of alcohol, etc. by . . . . . (specify date).

- Increase of . . .% in number of people with knowledge of common diseases and their control, e.g., diseases preventable by immunization, diarrhoea, diabetes, malaria, tuberculosis, leprosy, schistosomiasis, by . . . . . (specify date).

- Increase of . . .% in number of households with clean water by . . . . .(specify date).

- Increase of . . .% in number of community health workers making maintenance visits to water sites at least once a month by . . . . . (specify date).

- Increase of . . .% in number of households with latrines by . . . . . (specify date).

- Increase of . . .% in number of expectant mothers attending at least one antenatal clinic by . . . . . (specify date).

- Increase of . . .% in number of deliveries attended by health workers or trained traditional birth attendants by . . . . . (specify date).

- Increase of . . .% in number of eligible couples using contraceptives by . . . . .(specify date).

- Increase of . . .% in number of children under one year of age who have been fully immunized by . . . . . (specify date).

- Increase of . . .% in number of children under five who have growth cards by . . . . . (specify date).

- Increase of . . .% in number of cases of important local diseases (e.g., malaria) that are detected and properly treated; after a certain time a decrease will be expected as control measures take effect (specify time).

- Increase of . . .% in number of literate women by . . . . . (specify date).

- Increase of . . .% in number of contacts per capita with the health service by . . . . . (specify date).

Health infrastructure targets should indicate:

– health facilities and personnel;

– organization, including logistics;

– managerial arrangements, structure, roles, and responsibilities;

– target dates.

Here are some examples of health infrastructure targets:

Personnel

- Achievement of staffing norms in all facilities by . . . . . (specify date).

- Increase in numbers of dental assistants in health centres by . . . . . (indicate number) before . . . . . (specify date).

25

- Establishment of new cadres (indicate numbers and target dates).

- Revision of staff tasks by . . . . . (specify date).

- Organization of orientation courses on maternal and child health for all health centre staff before . . . . . (specify date).

- Organization of courses for community health workers and/or traditional birth attendants by . . . . . (specify date).

Health facilities

- Increase in number of clinics and health centres (specify number and target date).

- Establishment of laboratory services in health centres (specify target date and extent of improvement).

- Increase in number of facilities that are clean and well maintained (specify number and target date).

Logistic support

- Increase in number of vehicles and refrigerators that are in good condition and suitable for use the whole year round (specify number and target date).

- Increase in number of facilities that have essential drugs available throughout the year (specify number and target date).

Management

- Establishment of surveillance information system (records, maps, surveys, prediction of outbreaks) by . . . . . (specify date and extent of improvement).

- Intersectoral collaboration (specify target date and extent of improvement).

- Community participation in management by . . . . (specify date).

- Reduction in bypassing of health facilities (specify target date and extent of improvement).

Setting targets for health in Norway

In November 1985, a conference was held in Norway to discuss challenges to planning after the decentralization of primary health services to local municipalities. During this conference, the Minister for Social Affairs for the first time publicly declared Norway's commitment to the health for all strategy and also stated that the Government would prepare a national health plan.

Subsequently, the National Association of Municipalities, with support from the Directorate of Health and the Ministry of Social Affairs, prepared a series of conferences aimed at adapting the health for all policy to activities at the district level and providing the countries and municipalities with a new planning tool based on health for all principles.

The basic features of the national health policy are as follows:

1. Twelve problem areas have been identified on the basis of epidemiological studies; and twelve targets established accordingly:

    - to reduce inequities in health care
    - to develop and make use of health potential
    - to reduce the amount of disability
    - to reduce the incidence of specific diseases
    - to increase life expectancy
    - to reduce infant mortality
    - to reduce maternal mortality
    - to reduce mortality from diseases of the circulatory system
    - to reduce mortality from cancer
    - to reduce deaths from accidents
    - to reverse the upward trend in the suicide rate.

2. These targets cannot be achieved by work within the health system alone. Five areas of concern have been identified:

    - the health care system
    - life-styles
    - environmental risks
    - information and research
    - political support.

(Continued overleaf)

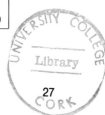

27

3. Six basic principles have to be kept in mind at all times to prevent contradictions within the system:

   – equity

   – community participation

   – health promotion

   – multisectoral cooperation

   – international cooperation

   – concentration on primary health care.

4. Within each area of concern there are specific objectives, the achievement of which will contribute to the realization of the ultimate targets. Three methods of work are common to all areas of concern, namely:

   – information

   – cooperation or network-building

   – resource allocation.

Within this framework, Norway has started a process of joint planning by the central authorities and the municipalities, and by health providers and health consumers. The process starts from the vantage point of the group targeted for improvement. It is at the local level that planners, health professionals, and members of the public need to decide which of the ultimate targets are most relevant to the health of the most important target groups, which areas of concern are most relevant, which are the most suitable partners in the venture, how to use information, how to allocate resources, and, finally, how to proceed.

KROMBERG, M. *Target setting and development of information systems in districts* (paper presented at an international meeting on Strengthening District Health Systems Based on Primary Health Care, Harare, Zimbabwe, August 1987).

Services required to achieve targets

Data from the analysis of the present situation in the district, for example, birth rates, death rates, and the incidence and prevalence of acute and chronic diseases, are necessary for a realistic estimate of the services required to meet such targets as the provision of antenatal care, maternity care, and immunizations. If the required information is not available, "guesstimates", based on a typical situation in a developing country, may have to be used. For example, using the figures below, the annual service workload in a district with 100 000 inhabitants, can be roughly estimated in terms of numbers of cases to be treated (Table 6):

- birth rate: 35 per 1000 population; pregnancies: 40 per 1000 (average of 3 antenatal visits);

- proportion of under-fives: 16% of total population (2 clinic visits per year);

- incidence of tuberculosis: 1 per 1000 population (1 clinic visit per month);

- annual incidence of episodes of diarrhoea: 2.2 per child under five (1 clinic visit per episode);

- annual incidence of acute respiratory infections (ARI): 2.0 per child under five (1 clinic visit per episode);

- normal deliveries: 80% of all births.

The content of services should be decided. For example, it might be decided that, besides weighing, the initial examination of children attending

Table 6. Estimated annual service workload in a district with 100 000 inhabitants

	New cases	Estimated clinic attendances
antenatal care	4000	12000
child care (under-fives)	16000	32000
tuberculosis	100	1200
moderate and severe diarrhoea in under-fives	35200	70400
moderate and severe ARI in under-fives	32000	64000
immunizations:		
BCG	3500	3500
DPT and polio (each)	3500	10500 (3 doses)
measles	3500	3500
normal deliveries	2800	2800

child welfare clinics for the first time should include screening for congenital abnormalities such as cataract, heart defects, descent of testes and congenital dislocation of the hip, depending on the staff deployed and the local importance of the condition. Discussions on the promotion of health in maternal and child health clinics might cover such topics as feeding, recognition of illness in a baby, family planning, and immunization.

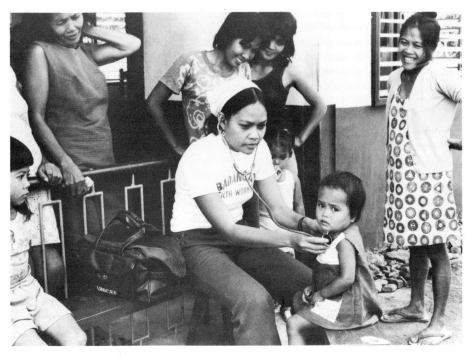

Home visit by a barangay health worker in the Philippines. *Photo WHO (20016)*

CHAPTER 5

The district action programme: improving health services

In a district action programme, clear instructions should be given regarding activities, targets, and resources for each category of work. The specific measures taken in a district will depend on the health objectives and service targets to be achieved. However, as services in districts are often organized into three broad categories—(a) curative, (b) maternal and child health, and (c) health promotion and the prevention and control of disease—it is worth considering what sort of measures might be employed in each of these areas. Limited resources will often dictate the implementation of just a few initiatives within each category of service, rather than complete coverage of all categories.

Curative services

For curative services to be adequate, appropriate facilities, trained personnel, equipment, and drugs must be provided for the key activities of diagnosis, treatment, follow-up, and referral. The ability to provide relief from pain and treatment for injuries is often the criterion by which people judge the health system. In addition, clean and tidy grounds, buildings, and staff create in the public a sense of confidence.

All population groups should have reasonable access, on a 24-hour basis, to medical services for acute and emergency cases.

The district health officer should ensure that relevant and simple books on the medical and surgical management of common conditions are available to health workers. He or she should also, particularly where such books are not easily available, issue documents and circulars giving treatment schedules for important or difficult conditions such as burns, acute diarrhoea, acute respiratory infections, malaria, tuberculosis, and leprosy. These will lead to a better use of drugs and improvements in the quality of care. An outline of the possible content of such schedules is given below, for diarrhoea and for burns.

- **Diarrhoea**. Mild cases: home treatment consisting of (a) giving plenty of locally available fluids to drink, such as rice water, fruit juice, or special home-made sugar and salt solutions; (*b*) increasing breast-feeding, where applicable; (*c*) continuing feeding, and watching for signs of dehydration. If dehydration occurs, the patient is treated with oral rehydration salts (ORS).

- **Burns**. Make a rough estimate of percentage of body burnt and depth of burns. If mild, treatment consisting of (*a*) administering analgesics, (*b*) protecting the site of the burn, and (*c*) reassuring the patient. If moderate or severe, treatment in health centre or hospital: (*a*) treatment for shock, may require intravenous fluids; (*b*) treatment of burn site; (*c*) penicillin injection; (*d*) referral for specific treatment. Severe cases may require specialized surgery.

Laboratory and radiological services can be of crucial importance in the diagnosis and treatment of patients. It is, therefore, important to ensure that adequate equipment and supplies as well as appropriately trained staff are available.

Much can be done to improve the rehabilitation of the disabled. WHO has developed a community-based approach designed to involve disabled people and their families in rehabilitation programmes through which they can be integrated into school, home, and working environments (*5*).

Strengthening the role of hospitals

The roles and functions of the district hospital can be summarized under the following five headings:

- Treatment of referred patients and emergencies.

- Coordination of health programmes. As well as treating individual patients, hospitals should be involved in the planning, coordination, implementation, supervision, and monitoring of primary health care in their respective catchment areas.

- Managerial and administrative support. Hospitals may be responsible for resource allocation and control throughout the district, depending on the way health services are organized in the country, for example, whether or not there is a separate health office to deal with administration.

- Education and training (see Chapter 7).

- Health systems research (see Chapter 9).

A WHO Expert Committee in 1985 drew up a list of 14 questions, reproduced below, to help hospitals re-examine their role in district health systems.

1. Does the hospital serve a specific population defined in terms of numbers, geographical boundaries or other characteristics?

2. Does the hospital view its responsibilities as extending to the population outside its walls?

3. Does the hospital consider its role in primary health care to include participating in the characterization of the problems, resources and needs of the population it serves?

4. Does the hospital consider it important to develop relations with all health agencies in the district, health practitioners of various types, community representatives, and authorities from other sectors in order to plan how the problems and needs of the population are to be dealt with?

5. Does the hospital participate in defining the prevalence and distribution of specific health problems (such as malnutrition, diarrhoeal diseases, complications of pregnancy, etc.), and help to plan who should be cared for outside the hospital and who should be hospitalized?

6. Does the hospital see its role as participating in the development and maintenance of an information system that would allow a continuous assessment of the status of major problems affecting the population, monitoring of programmes directed at those problems, and evaluation of their effectiveness?

7. Does the hospital see its role as participating in health manpower development throughout the area it serves, including helping in recruitment, training, supervision, and evaluation of health workers?

8. Does the hospital consider itself to be responsible for providing logistic support (such as bulk purchasing and storage of supplies, maintenance of equipment, etc.) to local health services in the surrounding district?

9. With respect to referral of patients, does the hospital consider its role to include developing the criteria for the referral of patients from peripheral health workers, specifying the information that should accompany patients to and from the hospital, and training the various personnel to ensure the effectiveness of such referral arrangements?

10. In viewing the overall costs of primary health care for the district, does the hospital consider it reasonable that resources should be allocated across institutional boundaries?

(Continued overleaf)

11. Does the hospital consider the assessment of the quality of care to be an important approach to evaluating hospital functions, and would the hospital consider it appropriate to extend this approach to primary health care services in the surrounding district?

12. Does the hospital consider it necessary to make specific functional and organizational changes within the hospital in order to accommodate or facilitate its role in support of district-wide primary health care activities?

13. In evaluating its own performance, does the hospital consider its contributions to surrounding primary health care activities as important components of its programmes? How would the hospital assess its contributions? For example, would it use perinatal and infant mortality rates for the whole district or the extent of coverage of the population as indicators of its performance?

14. Does the hospital consider it to be part of its role to join with community representatives and other interested parties in generating social and political support for the overall primary health care effort?

WHO Technical Report Series, No. 744, 1987 (*Hospitals and health for all*: report of a WHO Expert Committee on the Role of Hospitals at the First Referral Level).

Strengthening health centres

Besides a hospital or hospitals, a district may have smaller health facilities known by different names, including health centres, subcentres, clinics, polyclinics, group practices and dispensaries. They are distinguished from hospitals by the size of the population served, the types of service provided, and the categories of health problems dealt with. The term "health centre" is used here to include all facilities other than hospitals.

Nowadays health centres are operating increasingly on the principle of teamwork, whereby a patient may be seen by different health workers at different times. If this very efficient new approach is not to spell the end of personalized care, family cards and outreach programmes should be introduced by all health centres.

Important factors to be considered in strengthening health centres include:

- *The siting of health centres*, with accessibility as the key criterion.

● *The organization of services at the health centre.* Instead of arranging service days and opening hours to suit the staff of the centre, as is often the case, a health centre's opening days and hours should be determined in accordance with the needs, patterns of life, or life-styles of the community. For example, antenatal clinics could coincide with local market-days so that women can combine their antenatal care or family planning needs with their visit to the market. Also, health facilities should adopt the "supermarket" approach, i.e., provide the whole range of services, at all times, so that users do not have to make separate trips to the facility for each intervention.

● *The range of services,* which should include:

– curative care: examination and diagnosis, including simple laboratory investigations and treatment of common diseases, initial treatment of complex diseases pending referral to hospital. A few holding beds would be useful.

– follow-up treatment of cases referred back from hospitals.

– maternal and child health care.

– prevention and control of common diseases.

● *The interrelationships between health care personnel and the community.* The current training of health care personnel in many countries does not include teaching staff how to establish good public relations with the members of the community they serve. Yet everyone knows full well that the success or failure of a health centre mostly depends on this very ability.

● *Physical design of the facility.* The structure of a health centre should follow national guidelines, taking into account services to be provided, staffing, and availability of resources. Like the attitude of the staff, the design of the facility can improve or impair the acceptability of the centre. Both the outer appearance of the building and, to a greater extent, the internal lay-out should be related to, and in conformity with, the cultural environment of the community to be served. The same holds good for the waiting space and the treatment rooms. When organizing space, it is useful to start by asking two simple questions: What work is to be done here? Could this place be arranged in another way that would help the work and suit the patient better?

● *Availability of essential drugs and other supplies.* This must correspond to the prevailing patterns of health problems in the area.

- *Adequate response to community needs.* The activities carried out by the centre should be relevant to the priority health problems found in the particular community. This means that the health workers must be fully aware of the general health situation of the community they serve. They should learn to appreciate the type and extent of the community's health needs and know how to deal with them effectively, not only by using simple epidemiological methods, but also by ascertaining the opinions of the community.

- *Provision of affordable services.* In every country, the cost of health care is very much related to the health system as a whole and, in particular, to its planning and financing mechanisms. Hence, the overall financing mechanism of the country plays a determining role. Prohibitive costs to the patients will lead to the underutilization of available services, with inevitable repercussions on health.

- *Outreach services.* Provision of services outside the health centre premises is without doubt one of the key functions of a health centre. The development of such services is based on the realization that those who are able and willing to get to a health centre for care may represent only a small proportion of those who could benefit from the services it provides.

- *Adequate staff.* The services planned for the provision of care at a health centre will determine the categories of health worker included in the health centre team. To be able to provide basic services, the following workers (or their equivalents) should constitute the core of the team:

  - medical assistant (a few countries have physicians at health centres)

  - nurse/midwife

  - environmental health technician

  - laboratory aide or technician

  - health education/extension worker

  - statistical clerk.

- *Relationship with the hospital.* To ensure a viable referral system and good communication between the health centre and the hospital, the teams of both facilities should hold regular joint consultative meetings.

- *Training.* For health teams to be properly oriented to primary health care, it is important that student physicians, nurses, etc. who are undergoing training should have some contact with health centre activities during their basic, postbasic, and continuing education programmes. Also, community-based health workers should be trained both in the community and at the health centre, thus strengthening the links between the different types of worker.

- *Planning for health and evaluation of health care programmes.* The health centre is important in the context of intersectoral planning for health. The establishment of a management information system at the health centre level would supply the planning process for health with valuable inputs and also furnish indicators or tools for evaluating the various programmes of action at the health centre and community levels.

- *Learning by doing.* There is a need for studies on such important aspects of the health centre as coverage and quality of care. These should be carried out by all health centres, with certain centres selected to carry out more detailed studies, as necessary. The findings would then be used to improve the performance of health centres.

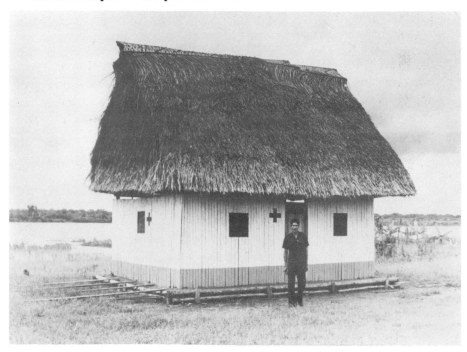

This rural health post in the Amazon basin of Peru typifies the first point of contact that many people have with "formal" health services. *Photo PAHO/J. Vizcarra (19944)*

Maternal and child health

Research has shown that action to improve the health of children and mothers will have a great impact on the health of the whole community. Maternal and child health services are concerned with preventive and curative activities at all levels of care.

Five types of activity can be identified:

- *Clinical services*—treatment of diseases.

- *Antenatal care.* Disease prevention and education are the main areas to be stressed. The identification of risk factors, such as poor weight gain, oedema, and hypertension, should be carried out on the basis of the history and of physical and laboratory examinations. A minimum number of visits should be prescribed for women with normal pregnancies. "At-risk" cases should be followed closely. Education should be provided at each visit, using presenters as well as posters and other printed material. Topics covered should include nutrition in pregnancy, breast-feeding, hygiene, labour, and family planning.

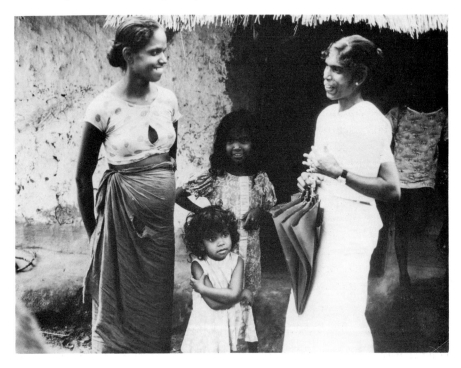

In India, a health visitor brings advice on family planning to the home rather than waiting for overburdened mothers to visit the clinic. *Photo WHO/J. Mohr (18264)*

- *Care of newborns and children*: the under-five clinic. The services provided include the maintenance of growth charts, health education (especially on nutrition), and immunization. There should be early identification and prompt referral of high-risk children, as well as those needing special services.

- *Family planning.* Family planning counselling is an important component of a maternal and child health service. Counselling should help women to choose contraceptive methods that are appropriate for their particular needs. Special attention should be paid to those at high risk such as adolescents and women who have had five or more pregnancies.

- *Health education.* Take the opportunity of every contact with patients to impart advice. Consider using demonstrations and discussion groups.

Maternal and child health clinics should aim at providing all five services at the same time so as to spare patients the hardship of repeated journeys. Rendering services more "humane" helps to make them more acceptable.

Maternal mortality

Every maternal death should be investigated and the findings used for improving maternal and child health services. The major causes of maternal mortality are haemorrhage, obstructed labour, abortion, eclampsia, and sepsis. Most of these deaths are preventable.

In deaths from haemorrhage, predisposing factors such as anaemia should be assessed. Was blood given in time? What was the blood loss at delivery? Were placenta and membrane complete?

Obstructed labour is a leading cause of maternal death and morbidity in the rural areas of many developing countries. Who attended the delivery? What was the duration of each of the stages of labour? It is often necessary to train traditional birth attendants so as to ensure that deliveries are attended by qualified workers. Besides improving their skills for safe delivery, training should enable traditional birth attendants to provide:

- antenatal care, including identification of high-risk women who should be referred to the health centre or hospital;

- education of mothers on better nutrition, the importance of breast-feeding, family planning, and management of diarrhoea, including the use of oral rehydration salts.

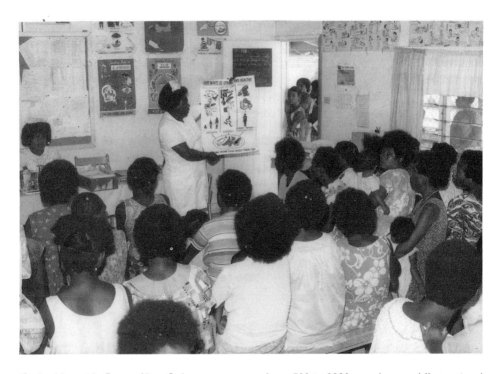

Each aid post in Papua New Guinea may serve from 500 to 3000 people, providing not only family planning advice but also outpatient treatment and health education. Here, a lecture on sensible foods for expectant and nursing mothers is in progress. *Photo WHO/J. Abcede (17745)*

One problem that often arises is the difficulty in reaching referral hospitals in obstetric emergencies, because of long distances and lack of means of transport. Local solutions to this problem must be sought, such as the establishment of waiting-houses near hospitals for expectant mothers at risk. Other solutions may be appropriate, depending on the main causes of morbidity and death from obstructed labour. Morbidity from obstructed labour, which includes fistulae and urinary incontinence, is in most cases a lifelong complaint.

In the case of death from abortion, the investigation should establish whether it was spontaneous or induced and, if induced, legal or illegal. In the case of toxaemia, it is particularly important to assess previous obstetric history and antenatal care. In the case of death from sepsis, details of the probable cause of infection should be established.

Perinatal and postneonatal mortality

The causes of deaths occurring between the twenty-eighth week of gestation and the first week of life (perinatal deaths) and those occurring between 1 and 12 months of age (postneonatal deaths) are similar. They include low birth weight (often due to maternal malnutrition), birth injury and asphyxia, and intrauterine or neonatal infections such as tetanus. However, there is an important difference: perinatal deaths are usually due to birth injuries and low birth weight. The perinatal mortality rate is therefore a good indicator of the quality of obstetric care. Infectious diseases are primarily responsible for postneonatal deaths. Improved maternal and child health services—in particular, better obstetric care and increased prevention of neonatal tetanus and other infections—can prevent many of these deaths.

School health

A school health programme should have four components:

- *Instruction in health.* As far as possible, health topics should be included in the teaching of other subjects. Teaching aids and materials adapted to the level of the pupils should be developed. Emphasis should be on primary schools, as there one is able to reach most children, including those from poor sectors, particularly girls, who are likely to drop out of further education.

- *Ensuring a healthy school environment.* This includes identifying deficiencies in the school environment and maintaining hygienic conditions, notably as regards cleanliness, housekeeping, and the disposal of liquid and solid wastes.

- *School health services.* These include the prompt diagnosis and treatment of disease. School health services should be part of the general health services.

- *Involvement of pupils in community health activities.* Such involvement could take different forms, including identification of major health problems, health education, sanitation campaigns, latrine-building, and other health-promoting activities.

The existence of a district school health committee, consisting of the district education officer and representatives of relevant sectors and agencies, will enhance the organization and management of school health programmes.

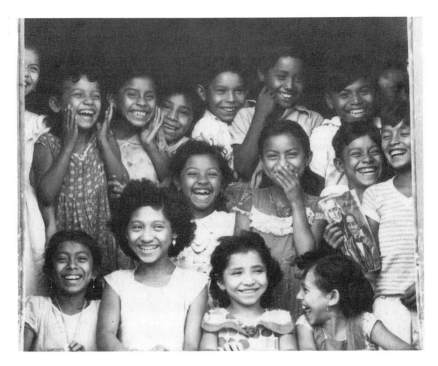

"Children's health, tomorrow's wealth"—happy schoolchildren in Mexico. *Photo WHO/ P. Almasy (8515)*

Health promotion, prevention and control of disease

The aim here is to encourage good health for individuals and population groups through health education and preventive activities. The preventive approach should permeate all aspects of district health work.

Health promotion

Further to the health education of individuals, which forms part of health care, health promotion can be carried out through folk media such as music, song, drama, dance, story-telling, and proverbs, as well as through radio, television, books, films, and games.

The most successful way of conveying health messages to the public is by involving the community itself. Thus, local composers, musicians, dancers, and comedians should be involved in developing appropriate health messages. Also, health workers can have discussions with local committees in order to gain an understanding of customs and traditions which will equip them to formulate appropriate messages in short stories or songs.

Communicable diseases

Actions for the prevention and control of communicable diseases can be divided into well-defined sets of activities which will vary in relevance depending on the specific disease:

- *Disease-specific activities* include the immunization of children and expectant mothers in maternal and child health clinics.

- *Case-finding and treatment* demand appropriate diagnosis and patient compliance. Mass treatment may be required in highly endemic areas e.g., where schistosomiasis is rife.

- *Vector control*. Several methods of vector control are possible, including the use of chemical insecticides and environmental measures such as swamp drainage. The development of vector resistance to various chemicals could be a big problem; expert guidance on the substance to be used should be obtained. A complementary approach to the control of vectors consists of direct community involvement in the elimination of domestic and peridomestic mosquito-breeding sites. In addition, personal protective measures to reduce contact between mosquitos and humans should be promoted.

- *Control of zoonoses*, such as rabies and brucellosis, by slaughter of infected animals, vaccination of animals, and control of milk and milk products.

- *Control of the environment* through safe water supplies, sanitary disposal of refuse, wastewater, and excreta, and adequate housing.

- *Promoting change in social and behavioural patterns*, e.g., identifying attitudes to disease prevention and immunization and behavioural patterns that increase the risk of falling ill.

- *Immunization* is the most cost-effective tool available for the control of certain major communicable diseases. Its value is enhanced if it is provided along with other preventive services that increase the chances of a healthy childhood and adulthood. Measures to achieve satisfactory coverage include ensuring community participation, outreach programmes, integration with other health service programmes, and continuous monitoring and evaluation, including the follow-up of those who drop out. To achieve high coverage it is important to use the education of mothers at antenatal clinics and of the public in general to promote enrolment of infants in child welfare clinics as soon as possible after birth. Secondly, it is necessary to set up an outreach programme to extend coverage to isolated families and to track down children who have missed appointments. The need for special efforts or campaigns to increase coverage should be carefully assessed. Such efforts may be useful if organized by the district as an extension of ongoing plans, rather than being a parallel one-off activity organized and managed centrally.

Epidemics

An epidemic is the occurrence of a number of cases of a disease, known or suspected to be of infectious or parasitic origin, that is unusually large or unexpected for the given place and time (6). To establish the existence of such an outbreak, an increase in the occurrence of cases compared with previous periods should be verified, using the data available. A graph showing numbers of cases over a period of time may be of use. It should be borne in mind, however, that a disease may sometimes be found in an area simply because of better diagnosis, and that, once a case is identified, others may be picked up as a result of greater awareness.

A disease is endemic when it, or its agent, is usually present in an area. An endemic disease may become epidemic when a non-immune population, such as newborn infants or migrants from non-affected areas, is exposed to the disease agent, or when climatic changes favour its proliferation.

Common sources of epidemics include foodborne diseases and infectious diseases such as cholera, plague, yellow fever, measles, dengue, viral hepatitis A, encephalitis, meningococcal meningitis, malaria, and African trypanosomiasis.

The investigation of an epidemic should establish the diagnosis of the disease, the source of the outbreak, and the mode of spread. The diagnosis can be established through a detailed clinical and epidemiological history supplemented by laboratory investigations. The history should establish **who** is affected (age, sex, occupation), with **what** symptoms (pain, fever, diarrhoea, etc.), and **when** and **where** the illness began. It is essential to try to establish the common characteristics of the group affected. A detailed history will lead to a provisional diagnosis, which will indicate what specimens should be taken for laboratory analysis.

Case-finding should focus on careful interviews and contacts. Once the symptoms and signs of the disease are known by the community, suspected cases may come forward. Knowledge of the incubation period of the disease may be helpful in tracing the source of infection. In a point-source epidemic, susceptible individuals are exposed to the disease agent at the same time. Most cases will, therefore, occur within a period of time reflecting the variation in the incubation period for the disease. The increase in cases is rapid, as indicated in Fig. 5. This type of outbreak is typical of water- and foodborne diseases, such as acute gastroenteritis. A vector-borne disease, such as yellow fever, may produce a point-source outbreak when a case enters an area harbouring the *Aedes* mosquito. Where a point source remains hazardous—for example, when contaminated food is eaten by different susceptible individuals over several days—cases will be spread over a long period.

In an epidemic of a contagious disease, in which the disease organism passes from one person to another, the increase in cases is gradual (see Fig. 6) by comparison with a point-source epidemic. The number of cases may

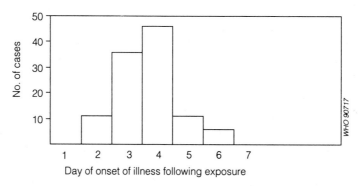

Fig. 5. Course of a point-source outbreak

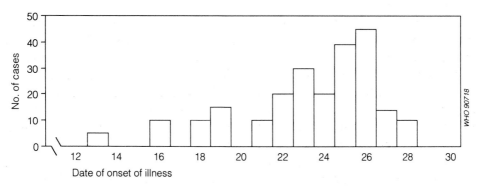

Fig. 6. Course of a contagious disease epidemic

decline with time as control measures are instituted or as the population acquires immunity.

During an epidemic, cases should be indicated on a map (with pins, for example), and the spread of the disease charted, in order to facilitate its control. Every effort should be made to identify lapses in environmental hygiene, such as poor sanitation, insanitary disposal of human excreta, inadequate food hygiene, or polluted water, that may be responsible for an outbreak. This information should then form the basis of measures designed to prevent the recurrence of the epidemic.

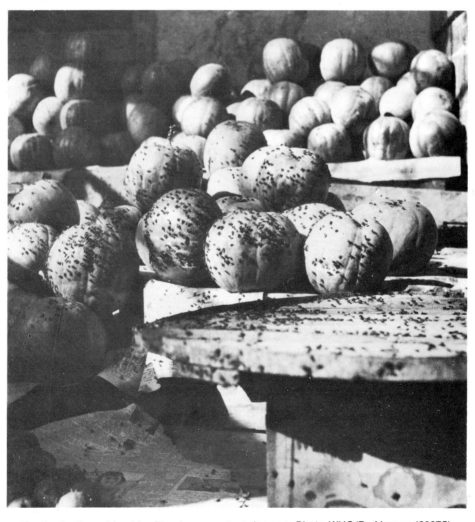

Contamination of food by flies is a constant danger. *Photo WHO/P. Almasy (20075)*

Management of epidemics

- Ensure that the district administrator and the ministry of health are kept informed and involved in the management of the epidemic. A district health or development committee can facilitate planning and coordinate action as necessary. Neighbouring districts should be informed of the outbreak. Meetings of staff dealing with different aspects of the epidemic should be organized regularly—if necessary, daily—to review the changing situation.

- Treat cases. Emergency accommodation in schools or elsewhere may have to be procured. Staff should be rapidly briefed on the treatment of cases and on personal safety measures.

- Isolate cases, if this is necessary to limit spread.

- Prevent spread by means of chemoprophylaxis (e.g., in the case of plague and malaria) or immunization (e.g., in the case of poliomyelitis and measles). Bear in mind that immunity takes about two weeks to develop following primary vaccination, but a shorter period following booster doses.

- Institute permanent preventive measures. These may include control of vector breeding, food hygiene (education and legislation), provision of safe water, and improvements in personal hygiene.

- Continue surveillance of the population to identify further outbreaks at an early stage, using such means as the notification of cases by local leaders, teachers, and laboratory staff.

- Prepare two reports on the epidemic: a simple shortened version for the public, and a more detailed account for the ministry of health and possible publication in a scientific journal.

Preparedness

Epidemics and natural disasters sometimes recur in defined areas and at particular times; some degree of preparedness is therefore possible. For example, areas that are susceptible to plague epidemics should have an active surveillance system to look out for danger signs.

A plan for dealing with outbreaks should be developed and should be known to health workers. A system of multisectoral coordination is indicated, as well as the training of staff for their role in the investigation and control of outbreaks.

Noncommunicable diseases

Chronic, noncommunicable diseases, such as cancer and cardiovascular diseases, are important causes of mortality and morbidity in the developed world. They are also becoming relatively more frequent in the developing countries with the adoption of Western life-styles and diet. The prevention of these diseases can no longer be neglected, particularly as the appropriate measures employ relatively simple technology and can be incorporated into schemes to prevent other diseases in the district.

The following approaches to the prevention of noncommunicable disease might be considered:

- *Clinical care*, e.g., taking blood pressure, diagnosing and treating diabetes, and counselling on smoking, diet, and alcohol abuse.

- *Health education* by means of printed materials, meetings, and the media.

- *Community organization*. This requires an assessment of the existing community organizations and their needs and aims. The cooperation of schools, women's organizations, the army, social welfare agencies, local newspapers, priests, and traders should be sought.

- *Environmental and structural improvements*. Smoke-free areas, low-fat food products, and salt substitutes should be promoted.

- *Other activities*. Measures could be undertaken for the control of cancer, cardiovascular diseases, accidents, and dental caries, according to their incidence and importance in the district.

Occupational health

The physical and social environment at the place of work can cause disease. Common hazards include dangerous buildings, machinery, dust, poisons, noise, heat, infections, radiation, and work stress. Accidental injuries to the head from falling objects and to the eyes, hands, and back (from incorrect lifting of heavy objects, for example) are fairly common. Other examples of preventable accidents are explosions, burns, and electric shock. Inhalation of small dust particles can lead to diseases such as silicosis, while cotton and asbestos fibres may cause respiratory ailments. Exposure to certain chemicals and allergenic substances can give rise to occupational dermatoses.

Exposure to repeated loud noise over a period of time damages the ear and can lead to deafness. Excessive noise also affects communication and efficiency at work.

The need to reduce costs with a view to greater competitiveness has led industries in some developing countries to apply lower standards of safety than those prevailing in developed countries, leading to relatively high accident rates. The number of road deaths is also much higher in developing than in industrialized countries.

In the course of their work, agricultural workers are particularly prone to certain infectious diseases such as anthrax, brucellosis, bovine tuberculosis, hookworm, and schistosomiasis.

The question *"What is your occupation?"* should feature prominently in discussions with patients and communities. The district health team should be familiar with the various occupations in the district, the diseases associated with them, and ways of preventing these diseases. A member of the district health team, possibly the person responsible for environmental health, could serve as a focal point for activities in this area. Working environments should be inspected regularly for risk factors, and discussions held with management and workers on measures to deal with any adverse finding. In large places of work, health and safety committees should be established.

A district occupational programme which would, among other things, ensure the availability of adequate skills to carry out the above activities ought to be developed.

Environmental health

In developing countries, environmental health should be considered together with occupational health, as the dividing line is rather thin: more often than not, industries are located in residential areas.

Important elements of environmental sanitation are: safe water supply, sanitary excreta disposal, disposal of solid wastes, drainage of surface water, safe food preparation, and shelter that is adequate from the standpoints of size and structural stability.

A protected water supply piped into individual dwellings or groups of houses may not be possible in the case of a large population, particularly in rural areas where households are widely dispersed. Alternative sources are springs, streams, ponds, lakes, surface wells, and deep boreholes. Action must be taken to find new sources and to ensure that these and others already

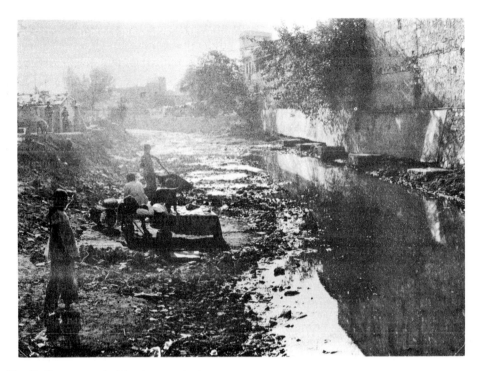

Hardly the most suitable place to do the weekly laundry: this sluggish stream is actually an open sewer. *Photo WHO/A. S. Kochar (18914)*

existing are protected by structural barriers against contamination. Treatment, usually by filtration, chlorination, or boiling, is often needed to ensure safety. Water may carry harmful bacteria and various protozoal and helminthic parasites. Periodic examination of water samples should be carried out to detect bacteria (the *Escherichia coli* count is commonly used in this connection). Involvement of the community, particularly the women, is essential in the planning and management of water programmes so as to ensure the continued maintenance of supplies and their correct use by the public.

Facilities for the sanitary disposal of human excreta are inadequate in many developing countries. Several types of latrine, at various levels of sophistication and adaptable to different environments, are available. The Blair latrine or ventilated pit latrine is so constructed that it is free from the flies and smell associated with ordinary pit latrines. Plans and targets for district action must be set up with the communities concerned (7). The support provided, e.g., subsidies for toilet slabs, will vary according to needs and resources.

The disposal of solid wastes is an increasing problem in the urban areas of developing countries because of organizational and financial shortcomings. Well-known technologies for the management of solid wastes are available (*8*).

Concerted action is needed to encourage and support communities in building houses that are structurally sound. The designs and materials used will depend on local conditions, particularly the climate and the level of development. Sensible siting can minimize the risks of flooding, landslides, road accidents, and exposure to noise and industrial emissions. Housing, village, and township planning committees should include competent health workers. Awareness of the importance of good, well-appointed houses, and of cleanliness in and outside the house, should be promoted through health education (*9*).

A suitably trained health worker should coordinate district activities in respect of food safety.

Mental health

Despite greatly expanded health facilities and personnel, mental health programmes remain rudimentary in many districts. Yet much can be done to prevent and treat the major problems encountered in this area, i.e., depression, suicide, epilepsy, schizophrenia, mental retardation, and behavioural problems arising from drug and alcohol abuse (*10, 11*).

The aim should be to raise the community's awareness of mental health issues and ensure that health workers and other leaders at all levels in the district have the basic skills and the commitment needed to support the programme. Guidelines based on national policies for the prevention and treatment of each of the more common conditions should be provided by the district health officer. These should cover diagnostic assessment, drug treatment, social management, and prevention of relapse.

The community health worker should be skilled in (*a*) the promotion of mental health, (*b*) the prevention of suicide, (*c*) the identification of major mental disorders, epilepsy, and alcohol and drug abuse, and (*d*) the management of psychiatric emergencies. He or she should also be able to advise and refer patients as necessary and to follow them up. The extended family provides care for chronically ill patients in many developing countries. The community health worker should accordingly work closely with community leaders and families.

Health centres should be able to provide simple treatment and/or sedation where immediate referral is not possible, and to continue treatment begun at the district hospital.

At district level, provision should be made for therapeutic care and mental health education. One of the physicians involved should have some skill in psychiatry. One health worker—a psychiatric nurse, if one is available—should be responsible for coordinating mental health work in the district. He or she should see that a sufficient stock of medicines is available, cooperate with workers in other disciplines and sectors, organize orientation courses for community health workers and community leaders, and support the health centre and the community health workers.

Outreach programmes

In districts in which the focus of health care is the local hospital or health centre, a major reorganization may be required in order to develop outreach programmes aimed at maintaining optimal health in the catchment area of the health facility concerned. Unfortunately, such programmes are often seen as being outside the work of the facility, or even as being in conflict with its interests.

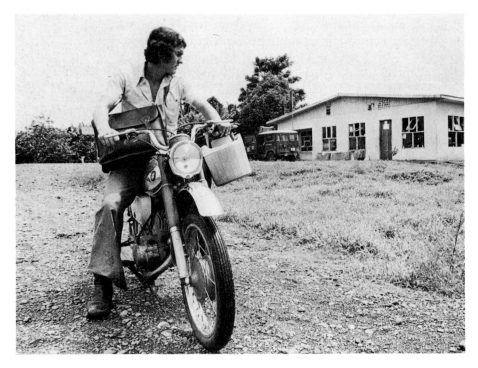

A rural health worker in Costa Rica arrives at the health post on his motor-bike—an essential part of his equipment in this rugged terrain. *Photo WHO/J. Littlewood (17896)*

This was probably justified in the past when many major rural health facilities in developing countries were manned by one person. It would have been unacceptable for the health worker to leave his or her patients, some of whom might require constant attention. The situation has improved dramatically in recent years with a considerable increase in the number of health workers and greater accessibility to curative services, so that responsibility can be accepted, not only for the sick, but also for maintaining health in a given geographical area. This approach has yet to be implemented on a national scale in many countries. Many problems have still to be overcome, but perhaps the most difficult is the inbuilt bias of health workers in favour of institution-based services.

The outreach programme's unit of care is the family and the locality (or localities) rather than the individual. Outreach programmes need to be planned by the district health team and may take different forms. They may be carried out by mobile clinics, either in public places or at health posts. The services provided are usually centred around maternal and child care. Here the activities include health education, antenatal care and care of children

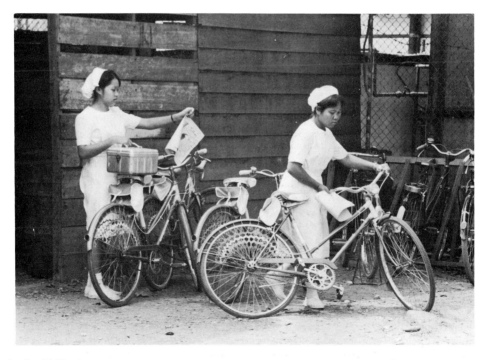

In the Philippines, nursing education is being reoriented to bring nurses closer to the real needs and problems of communities. This process is progressing slowly but surely, and the outlook is bright. *Photo WHO/J. Mohr (13957)*

under five, family planning, immunization, the provision of food supplements, chemoprophylaxis, and the treatment of common diseases.

Mobile teams consisting of full-time staff who travel to communities, bypassing local facilities, are costly and, in general, not advisable.

Canalización in Guatemala

Guatemala has a well developed countrywide system of health facilities, but people are reluctant to use them. A strategy to deal with this situation was introduced in 1984, based on what has been called *canalización*, i.e., a network of many "canals" branching out from the main "river of health care" and establishing links and lines of communication between health centres and communities.

The implementation of the strategy starts with a two-day seminar for professionals at the regional level. This is followed by a seminar in each district supported by the newly trained regional staff. At the end of the seminar, participants draw maps of the catchment area of each health unit, indicating houses, schools, paths, and water sources. This is divided into "sectors" consisting of the number of houses that can reasonably be visited by one member of staff—a nurse, midwife, or health inspector—within a 12-week period by devoting $1\frac{1}{2}$–2 days per week to this field work. Each sector is then divided into 12 zones.

At the beginning, each staff member does two things: he or she completes a simple census, and persuades one resident in each zone to be a "health collaborator". Priority is given to previously trained health promoters or traditional birth attendants. The health collaborators are trained before the first round of visits.

In each home, the staff member, appropriately kitted out and accompanied by the collaborator, performs the following tasks:

- raises awareness of health needs

- registers children under 5 for immunization

- gives instruction in oral rehydration

- makes referrals

- updates the census form.

As the programme gains momentum in a given district, other activities are gradually added: for example, dealing with acute respiratory infections, improving sanitation, growth monitoring, carrying out the first antenatal check, and advising on child-spacing.

On the day after the home visits, the staff member returns to the zone to perform the vaccinations planned on the first day. These are usually performed in the house of the collaborator who also goes to fetch any missing children. Those still absent at the end of the session are given an appointment for the following week in the next zone. On the afternoon after the vaccination session, the staff member visits the collaborator to review the activities and discuss any problems.

Results from this approach are encouraging: hospital mortality and the rate of hospitalization of children have fallen markedly, while coverage by immunization has risen dramatically. The utilization of fixed health services has also increased.

A gradual upgrading of the education of the health volunteers is contemplated. *Canalización* makes it possible to slant this upgrading towards the strengthening of overall community organization and development.

MONTOYA, C. *Development of district health systems in Guatemala based on primary health care*. Unpublished WHO document SHS 88/1 (available on request from Strengthening of Health Services, World Health Organization, 1211 Geneva 27, Switzerland).

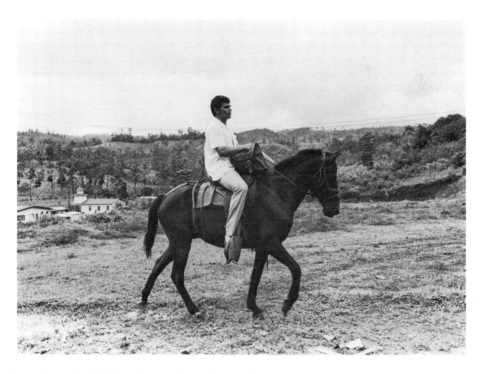

A health auxiliary doing his rounds on horseback in a rural area of Costa Rica. *Photo WHO/ J. Littlewood (18150)*

Ensuring quality services

Quality in health care is the degree to which the resources for health care, or the services included in health care, meet specified standards (*12*). All hospitals, health centres, and other health units should audit the quality of the services provided at least once every three months. The audit should be carried out by a committee chaired by the officer in charge at a session that may be attended by all staff. A record of the findings should be made for the information of staff who have attended the session and for future reference.

Quality is assessed on the basis of a review of charts and case-notes relating to various services (antenatal, child welfare, family planning and in-patient, for example). It is best to review the charts of one kind of service at a time. The charts to be reviewed are selected by some quasi-random method, e.g., every fifth chart, decided on the spot, taking into consideration the total number of charts. Where charts are few, it may be feasible to review all of them. It may also be decided to review all charts with particular features, e.g., all those relating to cases of maternal death.

The review will cover the adequacy of the clinical history, the examination, the investigations carried out, the management plan, and the instructions given. Below are some examples of areas to which attention should be paid.

Maternal and child health programme

- Are the scheduled activities of the maternal and child health clinic followed—for example, the provision of health education?

- Were the minimum prescribed procedures for pregnant women, e.g., blood pressure, urine, and haemoglobin checks, followed?

- Have abnormal findings, such as low haemoglobin or high blood pressure, been adequately followed up?

Any irregularities in individual records that may require further action should be noted.

The review will indicate the level of staff members' skills and knowledge, as well as gaps and lapses in the delivery of services. Such information is invaluable for assessing what further improvements are needed.

For quality assessment to be meaningful, there should be prior agreement on major issues relating to the way care is provided, e.g., criteria for admission to hospital, management of major diseases. Criteria for admission to hospital in pregnancy, for example, might include:

- severe anaemia

- persistent fever of more than 38.3°C (101°F) for more than 5 days

- abnormal findings in cerebrospinal fluid

- systolic blood pressure readings of under 80 mm Hg or over 200 mm Hg and/or diastolic blood pressure of less than 60 mm Hg or greater than 120 mm Hg

- onset of unconsciousness or disorientation

- bleeding

- chest pain and/or signs of acute ischaemia

- wound or surgical emergency

- obstetric problems, including obstructed labour.

CHAPTER 6

The district action programme: joint action

Community participation

Primary health care starts with the individual and the family. Action by individuals and by the community may bring about marked improvements in health and in progress towards the achievement of the district's health objectives and targets. In addition, the active involvement of communities in the planning and management of health programmes is essential to their success.

Individual and family action

Action for health by individuals and families may take the following forms:

- adoption of a healthy way of life
- prevention of specific diseases
- diagnosis and treatment of illness when it occurs
- appropriate use of available health services.

Of these, adoption of a healthy way of life and the prevention of specific diseases are the most likely to lead to a significant and sustained improvement in health.

- *Healthy way of life.* Individuals can limit or avoid certain risks to their health by adopting a healthy life-style based on such things as cleanliness and abstinence from smoking. It is better to start early so that habits adopted in childhood are carried through into adult life.

  Family planning is another healthy practice that can be adopted by individuals and families. Spacing births at least two years apart leads to better health for both children and parents.

  Healthy living not only entails behaviour that promotes the health of the body, such as eating sensibly, but is also concerned with behaviour that bypasses or limits the effects of health hazards in the community. A balanced diet is healthy, but its benefit may be limited if food and drinking-water are not protected against contamination. Hygiene and sanitation go hand-in-hand with proper nutrition.

- *Prevention of specific diseases.* Certain diseases may present such a threat to the health of a community as to demand a special effort by individuals and families to prevent them, or at least to reduce their frequency. For example, community members can help to control malaria by:

  - learning to recognize the symptoms of malaria and treat it with appropriate drugs;

  - making sure that family members take their prescribed treatments;

  - ensuring that expectant mothers, children under five, and others at high risk receive chemoprophylaxis;

  - taking measures to prevent mosquito bites: covering windows and doors with mosquito-proof materials, and wearing appropriate clothes;

  - taking measures to prevent mosquito-breeding: filling in pools of stagnant water, cutting long grass, and keeping the environment clean;

  - cooperating in national, regional, or local efforts to control malaria, e.g., providing samples for blood slides and cooperating in spraying dwellings with residual insecticides.

Community action

It is the responsibility of every member of the community to take appropriate action, not only because it offers an effective means of achieving a high level of health for all, but also because the failure of some individuals to participate can jeopardize the action taken by the others. For example, a single household with poor sanitation is a source from which infection can spread.

Communities may usefully take additional action as a whole or through particular groups such as schools, religious bodies, and voluntary groups. This includes:

- Clearing land for the construction of a health centre or road; making bricks and transporting materials to a building site; digging trenches for a piped water supply; clearing and tilling land for the production of nutritious foods. These activities could be carried out on a regular (say weekly) basis until the particular project is completed.

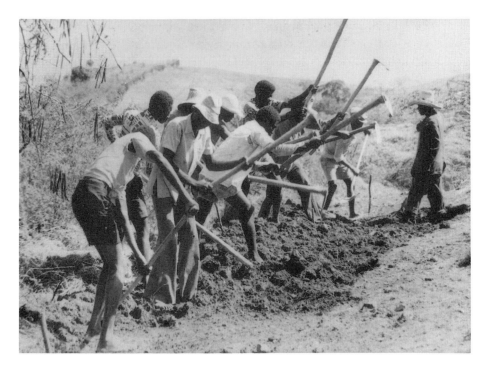

Involving the community is as important as political will for successful development measures such as improvement of water supply and soil conservation. *Photo WHO/FAO/ F. Mattioli (20017)*

- Educating the community about important health matters. This may be done through visits to individual households, a newsletter, or public events with an educational content, such as exhibitions, plays, and concerts.

- "Learning by doing". An example of this is the school production unit where pupils learn the skills needed for cultivating crops and vegetables, keeping livestock, and making and maintaining tools. The pupils' produce may be shared out within the community or put to more restricted use, e.g., to provide nutritious food for school or hospital meals.

- Collection of health and health-related data. Schoolchildren and community groups can play an extremely important role as collectors of information, preferably on a routine basis, in collaboration with the community health worker and other health staff. The data collected might include information on births, deaths, cases of sickness, nutritional status, levels of community sanitation and water supply, and immunization coverage.

- Participation in assessment of needs and in the identification of health priorities. Community representatives could be invited to attend meetings of the district health management team and thus become involved in decision-making.

Keeping the community informed

Communities need to be informed of how their activities are contributing to the achievement of district goals and targets, and how they compare with those of other communities in the district.

Possible means of doing this are as follows:

- Regular reporting of primary health care activities at meetings.

- Regular reporting of primary health care activities to individual families during household visits by the community health worker.

- Regular publication of a community "newspaper", which may consist of a blackboard set up in some public place, handwritten or printed wall-posters, or a printed newsletter distributed to households.

- Inclusion of news items about primary health care in the mass media—newspapers, the radio, and sometimes television.

Community health workers and leaders

Community health workers and local leaders have an important contribution to make to community involvement in primary health care. They represent the community and are responsible to it in carrying out their duties. They are also responsible for promoting changes in the community which will result in better health. They act as a link between the community and the health system, and are thus influential in helping the community and local health workers achieve mutual understanding and respect, thereby enhancing the effectiveness of primary health care. Community health workers can help achieve the fundamental goals of primary health care, that is, to make essential health care accessible to the entire population through a mixture of preventive, promotive and curative activities.

> ## Thailand
>
> Two types of village health worker are deployed in Thailand: village health communicators and village health volunteers. Village health communicators are trained and given guidelines to enable them to serve as disseminators of health information to groups of 10–15 families. For every ten communicators, there is one village health volunteer, who is given more training and responsibility in such areas as health promotion, disease prevention, simple medical care, and management. In Thailand today, there are about 42 325 volunteers and 434 803 communicators, effectively covering 90% of Thai villages (53 000 villages out of 57 398).

Mobilizing community resources

The resources available for health care, particularly in developing countries, are limited. Community involvement in primary health care makes it possible to mobilize community resources that might otherwise remain unused. Examples of such involvement are given below.

- *Action by the people.* This could include the provision of physical labour for building a health centre or constructing a safe well or sanitary latrine; the provision of transport to take a woman in labour or a sick person to hospital; the organization of a special day for immunization and for identification of children at special risk.

- *Provision of facilities.* A building owned by the community might be allocated to the community health worker for treating patients or storing medicines and records.

- *Provision of goods and materials.* The following could be provided: food such as grain, fruit, and fish for cooking demonstrations or for distribution to malnourished children; agricultural implements to boost community food production; or building materials, such as wood and bricks, to be used in self-help construction schemes.

- *Money or contributions.* Money donated for primary health care in a community may be used to purchase medicines, to purchase equipment such as agricultural implements, or to pay the community health worker.

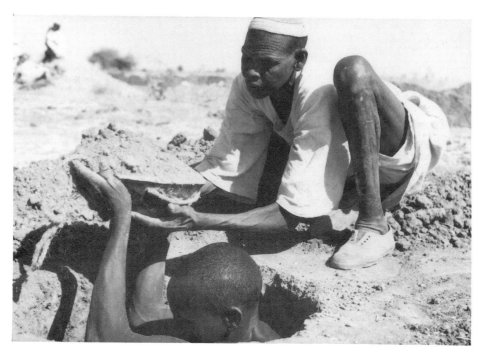

Digging for water is a community effort for these Sudanese villagers who are among the world's most desperately poor people. *Photo WHO/E. Schwab (9412)*

Methods of obtaining financial resources are many and varied; examples include:

- A fixed payment for each service provided.

- Payment for each service, depending on ability to pay.

- Payment that varies according to the type of service provided.

- Payment for drugs or a prescription, which may vary according to the type of drug and/or ability to pay.

- Payment through an insurance scheme, in which individuals or families make continued regular payments to provide for services when they are sick.

- Donations for services, the amount depending on the patient's willingness or ability to pay.

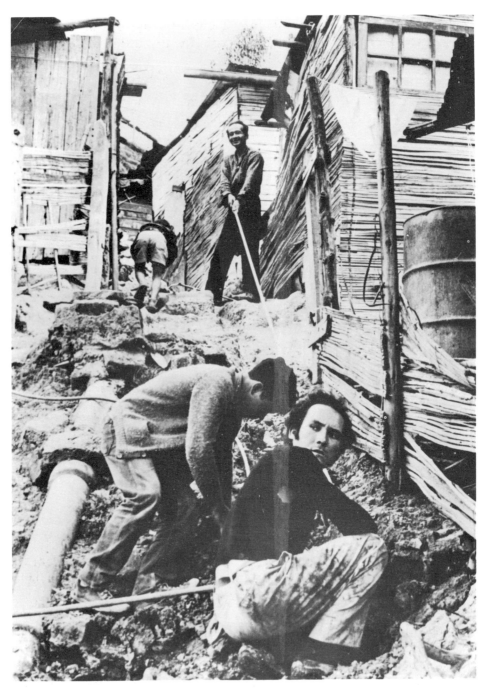

Health messages relayed to the public are motivating more and more communities to cooperate in laying water pipes and building latrines. *Photo WHO/UNICEF/H. Cerni (18909)*

– Payment through an insurance scheme covering preventive and promotive activities as well as individual illnesses in the community.

– Periodic donations (for example, by the local cooperative).

– Periodic fund-raising campaigns, which may include athletic or cultural activities organized by communities.

People's participation in Yugoslavia

In general, two forms of community participation may be distinguished. One consists in mobilizing people to participate directly in a community-based programme, by making contributions in cash or in kind or by offering their own labour; in this case, they are self-providers of services. The other involves the participation of users in the managerial process, so that they become decision-makers; in this way they are directly involved in the process of social control.

It is this second form of participation that has been developed in Yugoslavia in line with a more general strategy of promoting self-management in all public services and social activities. So-called "self-managing communities of interest" have a constitutional basis. Their assemblies comprise delegates of the health users (workers and citizens) and of the health providers. Within these communities, formed at all levels, health needs are identified, and programmes developed and managed, on a basis of solidarity. There is a free exchange of labour between the users and the providers of health care.

Community self-help schemes

In many countries, work schemes undertaken by communities on a self-help basis have made important contributions to development. Apart from the construction of health facilities, possibilities include the improvement of community housing and the construction or maintenance of (*a*) wells and boreholes providing safe drinking-water, and (*b*) facilities for the disposal of excreta and wastes.

The term "self-help" has been taken to mean that a community takes complete responsibility for a project from planning through to implementation, including the provision of all resources. In practice, resources such as building materials and other equipment are often obtained from outside authorities. To ensure effective use of the community's resources, it is

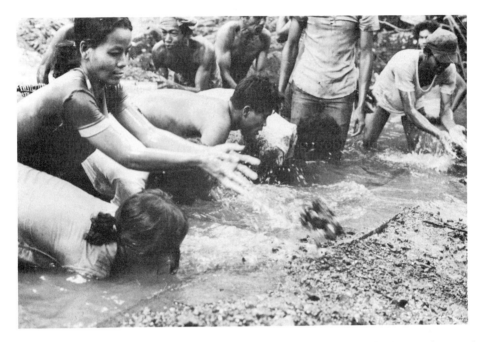

Twice a month, the villagers of Sarawak spend a morning at the watershed removing sand, gravel, and silt and generally cleaning up the dam. *Photo WHO/J. Abcede (17112)*

essential that good cooperation should be established between the community and all relevant outside authorities, from the earliest stages of planning to completion of the project.

Bottom-up planning

Emphasis should be given to the development of programmes through dialogue with the community, rather than using a top-down approach, whereby communities are expected to implement projects that have been developed at higher levels or even outside the country. Village committees, women's and youth organizations, and similar bodies may need to be set up to facilitate the necessary participation. Joint work with communities calls for attitudinal changes on both sides and is a slow process. It can be achieved once communities develop and take their health and their lives into their own hands to a greater extent.

Thailand: "Basic Minimum Needs" strategy

Community participation in top-down programmes usually consists of contributing labour and resources. The community's understanding of a problem is seldom considered, nor are there mechanisms to communicate such information upwards. To redress this situation, Thailand has adopted the Basic Minimum Needs strategy, which is essentially a data-collection exercise carried out by village leaders supported by government officials. There are eight basic minimum needs:

1. Family members should consume sufficient nutritious and safe food to meet their physical needs.

2. Every family should have appropriate shelter and enjoy appropriate environmental conditions.

3. People should have ready access to those basic social services that are necessary for maintaining life and activity.

4. People should enjoy security as regards their lives and possessions.

5. There should be efficient production and procurement of food for all.

6. Families should be able to plan the spacing and number of their children.

7. People should participate in developing their own and their community's way of life.

8. People must be able to pursue their spiritual development.

Zambia: district action committees for primary health care

In 1985, a national group, with members drawn from the Ministries of Health, Agriculture, Labour, and Social Services, as well as the National Food and Nutrition Commission, the Institute of African Studies, and the Department of Community Medicine at the University of Zambia, was formed to provide support for a project to strengthen intersectoral action in a number of selected areas, starting in Mumbwa District. Apart from developing and sustaining intersectoral initiatives in the district, the project was intended to give members of the national primary health care committee and the district committee an opportunity to gain first-hand experience of carrying out community diagnoses and engage in a dialogue with members of the community, and also to bring the national group into closer contact with concerns and constraints at the district level.

Three days of orientation training were organized for the district primary health care committee by the national action group. The subjects reviewed included primary health care strategies in the district, the rationale and importance of intersectoral action in health development, and the details of the project. The district committee identified three areas in which the project could be initiated. Local committees were formed in these areas, and planning for community diagnoses went ahead. The plans included the development of a household questionnaire by national, district, and local committee members. In early 1987, household surveys were conducted in the three selected locations. National participation was gradually reduced so that the final survey was conducted mainly by the district team. The data are now being analysed and will be used by the district committee in discussions and planning sessions with the local committees.

Intersectoral action

The district health system should be concerned with improving the health and quality of life of the population, and not just with providing services for the care of the sick. However, the efforts of the health sector alone are not enough to bring about significant improvements in health. Other sectors such as economic development, agriculture, education, and water supply may, in some situations, have an even greater potential for improving health than the health sector itself. In trying to achieve their individual sectoral objectives, they exert a powerful influence on health, both positive and negative.

The district is in a better position than the province or the central authority to achieve effective coordination with health-related sectors in the planning and implementation of health development. A key step in strengthening district health systems is to ensure intersectoral action.

Approaches for encouraging intersectoral action include the following:

- When planning new initiatives, greater emphasis should be placed on risk factors for health rather than on actual health problems. This will naturally lead to intersectoral action, since the reduction of many risk factors does not necessarily fall within the sphere of the health sector itself but may depend on other sectors. For example, achieving cleaner water supplies is a task for the district council's utilities department, while action to improve knowledge of health issues, such as family planning, nutrition, and the dangers of smoking, may quite reasonably be taken jointly by the education and health sectors.

- Initiatives to reduce inequities in the health sector may lead to intersectoral collaboration. This is because such inequities are closely linked to inequities in other sectors such as income, nutrition, water supply, sanitation, and education.

- Intersectoral collaboration may be fostered through the administrative structures at district level. At this level, senior health service staff will be well known by the local community and should be able to participate in the proceedings of district development committees, municipal councils, etc. and influence them. Special intersectoral boards may also be formed to promote intersectoral activities. In addition, district health staff can approach district committees responsible for other sectors, e.g., the local education committee.

- It might also be advantageous to select or appoint district health staff who would have special responsibility for the promotion of intersectoral cooperation.

Some examples of contributions to health development by specific sectors are described below.

Agriculture

Widespread malnutrition is rampant in many districts in developing countries. The adoption by governments of appropriate agricultural policies, relating, for example, to food prices, land ownership, and locally cultivated crops, is crucial in ensuring an adequate supply of nourishing food. Targets should be agreed upon and set with regard to the supply of good food and nutritional status (for example, weight for age and birth weight). Activities that can help ensure a sufficient supply of nutritious food include: assisting the community, through modern methods of farming, to increase food production; improving grain storage and preservation to reduce losses; and finding markets for farmers' products.

Rural development

Experience shows that overall economic development contributes to improvements in health. Local income-generating projects should be promoted and supported.

Women's affairs

The role of women, as both providers and receivers of health care, is being increasingly recognized. Women's organizations should be involved in planning and managing health programmes. These organizations can encourage women to practise family planning and breast-feeding, educate mothers to attend maternal and child health clinics, and inspire them to educate their children to observe personal hygiene.

Education (formal and informal)

The success of health programmes is related to literacy rates, particularly among women. For example, infant mortality is lower in countries or districts where the literacy rate among women is comparatively high. District programmes should, therefore, encourage widespread improvements in formal and informal education, particularly education of women.

Water and sanitation

Targets should be set, and programmes developed and implemented, for the provision of safe, potable water and for the sanitary disposal of excreta.

Housing

Many people, particularly in urban slums and in rural areas, live in substandard dwellings with little space and ventilation. Such conditions are conducive to the spread of airborne diseases. District plans for improving dwellings should be encouraged.

The integrated service post in Indonesia

In Indonesia, community health services are available from integrated service posts called *posyandu*. There volunteers from the community and regular staff from the health centres come together for one day each month to offer integrated family health services.

The *posyandu*, or integrated service post, is a centre for communication and the delivery of health services by and for the community. It aims

---

at integrating:

- intersectoral development programmes

- intrasectoral health programmes

- professional and traditional services.

The health services provided by the *posyandu* cover maternal and child health, family planning, immunization, improvement of nutrition, and diarrhoeal disease control.

The *posyandu* is organized and supported by the Women's Family Welfare Movement (PKK), a voluntary movement whose goals are the development of communities, both in rural and urban areas, and the promotion of better welfare and a decent standard of living. The movement's target is the family unit, with the mother as the focal point. The PKK is part of the programme of the Community Resilience League which is concerned with community participation in the execution of rural development policies and helps plan and implement local development activities.

The PKK and the Community Resilience League have boards at all levels of local government and at the national level. Throughout the country, PKK teams facilitate, motivate, monitor, and supervise the movement's activities at the next lower level. The lowest level is called the Group of Ten and consists of ten households served by one PKK member. The process of community involvement is usually as follows:

- At a meeting of official and unofficial leaders, held at village level, health centre staff introduce the concept of the integrated service post.

- The community, with support from health centre staff, conducts a community self-survey with the objective of identifying problems and increasing awareness of health needs.

- The results of this survey are presented and discussed at a "community consensus meeting", in which the whole community participates. During this meeting priority problems and solutions are determined.

In areas where the *posyandu* is well established, community volunteers (preferably accompanied by the local chief) visit the homes of target groups one to two days before the *posyandu* session. After the session, a meeting is held to discuss the effectiveness of the preparations, the implementation of the session, and the coverage achieved, and to complete the recording and reporting of the day's activities.

The *posyandu* strategy is still evolving and requires strengthening. A recent development is that of rewarding the *posyandu* for identifying illiterate mothers of under-fives. These mothers are then offered literacy training and informal guidance on home industry. Other health-promoting activities are being explored.

Integration of vertical programmes

The great technological progress seen in the 1940s and 1950s, particularly the development of vaccines and more effective drugs, led to the initiation of various special programmes aimed at particular health problems. Many campaigns were organized against communicable diseases such as malaria, smallpox, sexually transmitted diseases, yaws, tuberculosis, and schistosomiasis. Through the vertical approach, substantial advances were made in the control of a number of diseases, and it undoubtedly contributed to the considerable improvements in health observed over the past 20–30 years. The eradication of smallpox is a noteworthy example. However, not all positive results are attributable to specific campaigns. If yaws, for instance, was eradicated in a number of countries in the 1950s by special campaigns, it disappeared from many other countries around the same time, probably as a result of improved hygiene, housing, clothing, water supplies, and health services.

From the perspective of the community, the trouble with vertical programmes is their fragmentary approach to community health. The early 1970s saw renewed emphasis on integration. In nearly all vertical programmes, experience has shown that the effective coverage of large populations where services are limited demands a health infrastructure in continuous contact with individuals and families. Such an infrastructure requires: a network of facilities, manpower, supplies, and transport; an information system responsible for surveillance of diseases and populations and capable of monitoring progress; manpower development, including training and supervision; and managerial capability, notably in planning and evaluation.

Priority in the development of primary health care should, therefore, be given to building the requisite infrastructure alongside associated programmes. The participation of outside agencies, which promote vertical programmes simply because they can obtain quick results that will be visible to their governing bodies, may be counterproductive. It should be possible to arrive at a compromise whereby the agencies would support the overall development of the infrastructure, as well as individual programmes.

Integration faces many problems. Where there has been a history of strong vertical programmes using various categories of single-purpose worker, there may be difficulties in adjusting differential salaries, seniority levels, etc. The attitude of health workers may also be a problem: often staff are not psychologically prepared for change, continue to give preference to their previous programmes, and fail to create the desired linkages across primary health care programmes.

District health officers should be aware of these difficulties and constantly review the organizational structure and managerial procedures in order to alleviate the situation. The joint training of staff and regular meetings may be of help.

It is inevitable that, in certain circumstances, the generalist will have to depend on the expert for guidance. The presence of specialized units at various levels of the ministry of health may be necessary to deal adequately with particular situations and to determine and monitor appropriate forms of health action.

At district level, the district health officer is solely responsible for the execution of all programmes within his or her area of jurisdiction. The district health planning or management team must not be bypassed, and all activities should be carried out through the member of the team responsible for the activities indicated in Fig. 7.

The distribution of financial responsibility for the various programmes has been a bone of contention in a number of countries. While specialized technical units at the central level certainly may need a clearly defined budget for the support they provide, they should not as a rule have financial responsibility for routine district primary health care activities. The budget for operational activities should be the responsibility of the health team at district level.

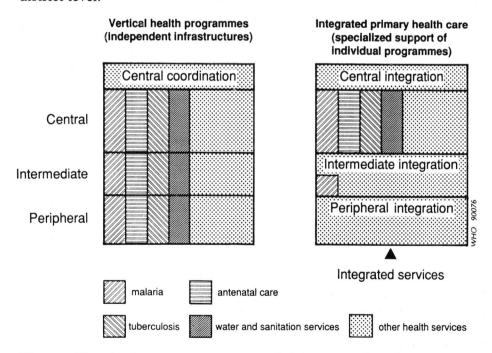

Fig. 7. **Vertical programmes and integrated primary health care**

Finally, the district health team needs to bear in mind that the ministry of health is often only one of several organizations providing health services in a district. Nongovernmental organizations and government departments, particularly those responsible for local government, operate extensive health care programmes. In addition, it is necessary to consider both private and traditional practitioners, not to mention self-medication, which may occur on a large scale. Private spending on health in some countries is 4–5 times greater than public spending on health. Useful and effective traditional practices can be included in, or coordinated with, organized health care. The work of traditional midwives has been closely linked with maternal and child health in many countries, and there is little controversy about their role. The situation is different, however, with other traditional practitioners. A number of countries have introduced elements of traditional medicine into the curricula of health workers and aspects of western practice into traditional medicine; traditional practice has thus been incorporated into formal, organized care. But in some countries, there is considerable hostility between the two systems. In all communities, traditional practitioners are influential figures to whom people turn for advice, openly or in confidence. The type of linkage or coordination between the two systems will vary according to circumstances in the district and national policies. The organization of orientation meetings for traditional practitioners (on their own or with other local leaders) will facilitate collaboration. Coordination with relevant agencies is crucial for the success of primary health care, and it is useful to have some kind of medium — for example, a biennial or annual meeting — for the exchange of ideas and the development of joint plans with major health agencies.

Achievements of an integrated programme in Sri Lanka

In an attempt to strengthen the delivery of primary health care, Sri Lanka has improved the organization and management of its district health systems and avoided vertical programmes and campaigns. For example, Sri Lanka does not have a separate immunization programme; immunization is an integral part of the maternal and child health programme.

This is the context in which the results of the 1986 review of the immunization programme, carried out by Sri Lanka with the help of WHO and UNICEF, should be seen. Over 90% of the children surveyed were found to have received BCG and three doses of diphtheria/pertussis/tetanus (DPT) and oral poliovirus vaccines. The high levels of coverage exceed those found in many developed countries.

CHAPTER 7

Implementation

To strengthen district primary health care, it is essential to improve operational management. This chapter presents six key issues pertaining to good management.

Personnel and training

The types of personnel required in a district will depend on the local situation. What is important is that the level of manpower and skills is matched with the tasks to be carried out, and that the staff are adequately distributed throughout the district health system. In many countries, staffing levels are adequate, but further training may be required in order to reorient them towards primary health care.

Staff are often ill-prepared for the changes required by current health training programmes. Moreover, the need for intersectoral planning will demand readiness on the part of health workers to adopt new ways of thinking and interact more widely with communities and other development sectors. It is therefore crucial to ensure appropriate orientation of the district health team, perhaps by means of annual or biennial one-day seminars with members of the district development committee. The support of the regional or central level in organizing such seminars should be sought.

Many health workers, particularly in peripheral units, work in isolation. Some may not have attended refresher courses since qualifying, perhaps many years earlier. Their skills, which begin to decline after qualification, may sink to a level where they are not only useless but an actual hazard. Sometimes workers are overtrained, with the same people attending courses that are usually related to one programme only. A plan of action for the reorientation of all health staff within the district may need to be developed, and the potentials of activity-based and distance learning explored.

Activity-based learning combines in-service training seminars or workshops with regular supportive supervision. An initial workshop introduces new skills, which are then implemented in practice with supervisory support. The problems encountered may be discussed at a second workshop several

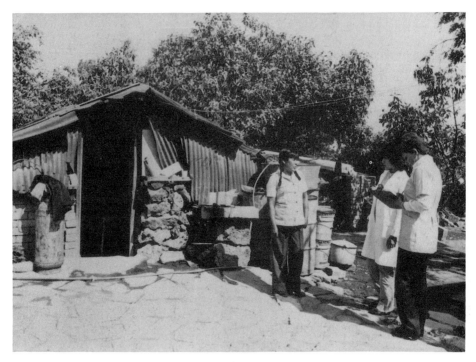

Medical students in Mexico must undertake work in local communities before they can qualify as doctors. Here two students visit a patient in a rural Mexican community. *Photo WHO/Mexican Ministry of Health and Welfare (19225)*

months later. A further period of implementation is followed by an assessment workshop.

The principles underlying district health systems, as outlined above, have considerable implications for the type of training and orientation that should be provided. Training should impart epidemiological knowledge and skills that will enable health workers to work out the rationale behind what they do and plan their work to the best advantage. For example, they will know when to expect malaria or diarrhoea in their area and thus be able to plan appropriate preventive and curative activities. The often expressed fear that peripheral workers are being asked to do too much stems from a failure to realize that, if properly oriented, peripheral health workers can be their own epidemiologists.

A problem that many district health officers have to face, therefore, is that of coordinating individual training courses for programmes such as immunization, the provision of essential drugs, and the management of diarrhoeal diseases, tuberculosis, leprosy, etc. The training materials for these

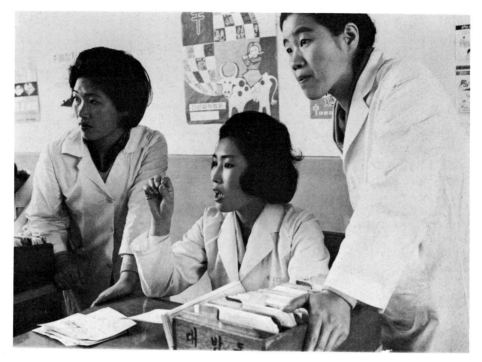

A nurse from the Korean National Tuberculosis Association explains to two student nurses how to interview patients and take case histories. *Photo WHO/P. Boucas (10780)*

programmes have usually been prepared separately. Various ways of integrating the training have been and continue to be explored by individual countries and by WHO. Important health problems for which no specific manuals have been proposed may also need to be identified and dealt with in training courses.

Training *awraja* health managers in Ethiopia

The strengthening of district health systems requires dynamic leadership and continuous attention to management. Strong interlevel links, intersectoral coordination, and community participation in primary health care are all vital to the effective management of a decentralized infrastructure. The training and responsibilities of health personnel, however, often limit their ability to attend to these factors. In 1986, Ethiopia accordingly decided to introduce a new type of professional health worker—the *awraja* (district) health manager—to redress the situation. A two-year training programme for graduate physicians was

---

introduced, combining theory, field experience, and in-service super-vision.

The training of medical graduates as district health managers in Ethiopia is a first attempt to develop leaders and agents of change for the district. The new course has been designed with the aim of training a new brand of primary health care manager to meet the needs of the *awraja* health administration. These managers are expected to be much more than administrators. They have to be leaders, trainers, and a source of inspiration as regards the development of primary health care.

In contrast to traditional curricula, the training programme for *awraja* health managers is competency-based, due account being taken of the job description.

Awraja health managers will:

- work with mass organizations in the *awraja* to identify health-related problems and advise on means of overcoming them;

- organize, manage, and administer the health services of the *awraja* so as to ensure maximum coordination of the available services and to achieve optimum coverage, efficiency, and effectiveness;

- plan the health services in the *awraja*;

- ensure the coordination of intersectoral health-related activities;

- develop and/or strengthen the system for the collection, analysis, and interpretation of information necessary for health planning and management, including monitoring and evaluation at all levels in the *awraja*;

- participate in the planning and operation of training programmes for professional and other cadres of health staff in the *awraja*.

Above all, the training stresses the importance of the *awraja* health manager as an agent of change. Through discussion, persuasion, and mobilization, he or she must bring about a commitment to primary health care on the part of professional health workers, members of other key sectors, and the mass organizations involved.

In order to impart the knowledge and develop the skills needed to carry out these functions, the course emphasizes the concept of "learn-ing by doing". The first part of the course consists of theoretical training in planning, epidemiology, management, and communication, inter-spersed with two months of practical field work, with emphasis on designing surveys involving the community and on the identification of priority problems.

During the following year, the students become acting *awraja* health managers and are expected to put into practice what they have learned. They also undertake a research project which forms the basis of their dissertation leading to an MSc degree in community health.

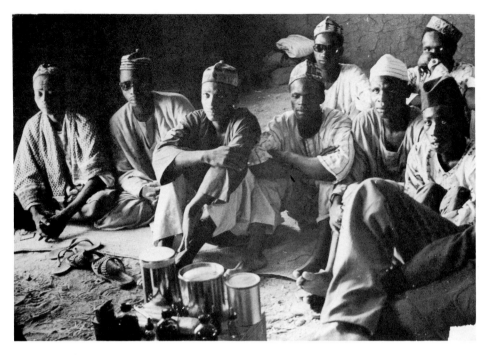

Village medical helpers attending a course on primary health care in Torodi, Niger. *Photo WHO/R. da Silva (17213)*

National and district authorities may also consider starting primary health care newsletters, where these do not already exist. Many countries are finding such newsletters very useful for the continuing orientation of staff and the exchange of ideas. The installation of district and health centre libraries is also an important cost-effective way of ensuring continued learning and one that remains surprisingly neglected both by governments and international organizations.

The district should also train new community health workers and traditional birth attendants as the need arises. The latter play a most important role, for not only are 60% of all babies in some developing countries delivered by them, but they are also actively involved in child care (growth monitoring, nutrition education, prevention and treatment of diarrhoea, immunization, etc.) and family planning. Hence, careful consideration must be given to the content of their training. For example, it is important to ensure that they are able not only to carry out deliveries safely and cleanly, but also to detect abnormal conditions in the antenatal and postnatal periods and make appropriate referrals. As to the place for training, should this be a hospital, a health centre, or the village? Insistence on training traditional

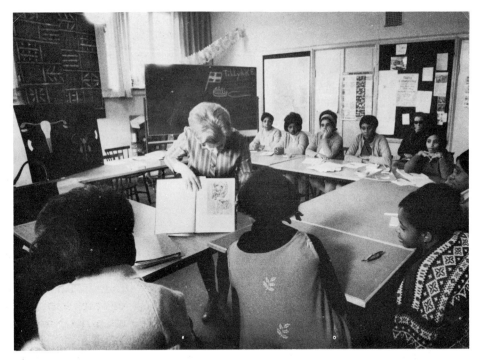

Course on family planning for preschool and kindergarten teachers from developing countries. *Photo WHO/E. Mandelmann (15551)*

birth attendants in hospitals, where they are made to wear such things as masks, aprons, and boots, has tended to institutionalize them. Also, communities may feel that, after such training, the remuneration of the birth attendant is no longer their responsibility but that of the ministry of health. This usually happens when, on returning from their orientation course, traditional birth attendants take it upon themselves to double, or even quadruple, their "expected" remuneration. This said, some training must nevertheless take place in a health facility so as to include supervised attendance at deliveries.

The district may also have to organize training and/or orientation programmes for special groups. Workshops on the subject of primary health care and the school need to be organized for schoolteachers in the districts, and should be planned in close cooperation with the district health education officer and the ministry of education.

Finally, the health staff need to organize orientation and/or mobilization activities for community leaders, youth movements, women's organizations, political parties, trade unions, and communities in general. These can be varied: workshops, films, district health weeks, etc. Where district health teams have worked closely with other leaders, innovative and effective programmes have been developed. One such was the founding by a governor in a South Asian country, on the occasion of a religious feast, of a "healthy life" movement, whose objectives were "small, happy and prosperous families; the reduction of infant and child mortality, and of the crude birth rate, through integrated interventions in maternal and child health, nutrition, family planning, immunization, diarrhoea control, and improvement of environmental health."

Organizational structure

To achieve planned targets more easily, it might be necessary to change the organizational structure of the services and to link service and managerial functions.

In some countries, public health and curative functions at district level are administered independently in separate units, namely the health office and the hospital. However, in an increasing number of countries both these units come under the district health officer, who is based in either the hospital or the health office. If the administration is hospital-based, the danger is that it may be hospital-dominated, though it would also offer some advantages,

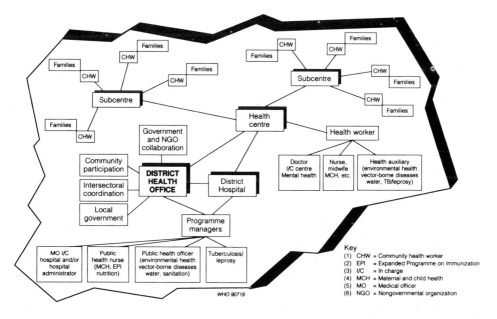

Fig. 8. Example of district organizational structure

including greater potential for mobilizing hospital staff for community programmes.

Organization at the subdistrict level (i.e., at the health centre and subcentre levels) will vary from country to country, depending on the numbers and types of staff deployed and on differences in health needs. The staffing pattern of peripheral health facilities will also vary greatly. A question that often arises is whether or not to use multipurpose workers. In sparsely populated areas, a multipurpose worker is preferable, whereas, in densely populated areas, it may be more efficient to have specialized workers.

Fig. 8 provides an example of an organizational structure found in some countries. This structure facilitates the comprehensive implementation of primary health care. The services are divided into three categories: (1) curative, (2) maternal and child health (including immunization and nutrition), and (3) preventive (including environmental health, water supply, and infectious disease control).

The district primary health care team

The district health management team might include the district health officer, a hospital doctor, a public health nurse, a public health inspector, a hospital administrator, and a finance officer. Each health facility will probably also have its own team. Other teams in a district may include health centre and/or hospital advisory boards, and committees for school, village, or district (health) development (see list below). The community should be adequately represented on these boards and committees. It is important to ensure that the tasks of the teams are clearly defined and oriented towards the achievement of district health objectives.

The following is a list of the various health teams that might be found in a district (average numbers in parentheses):

District (health) development committee (1)

School health committee (1)

District health management team (1)

District hospital advisory board (1)

District hospital management team (1)

Health centre/subcentre advisory board (30)

Health centre management team (30)

Village (health) development committee (60)

Effective use of team members

Experience shows that a number of health care workers are capable of doing much more than they are doing at present. For example, with proper motivation and guidance on primary health care, the health inspector could play a leading role in the improvement of environmental sanitation and the provision of safe water. The peripheral midwife, the mainstay of maternal and child health care in many countries, with simple training could play a greater role in educating communities on how to avoid disease and on healthy life-styles.

More important still are the staff of nongovernmental organizations. Countries are for ever "discovering" lay or religious associations, youth clubs, or women's groups which turn out to be of the greatest assistance in the achievement of district health targets. Also, in many countries, church organizations train and employ as many health workers as the ministry of health. Team-building would greatly benefit from a good analysis of the staffing situation and from a proper allocation of tasks.

Leadership

Leadership means influencing others so that they achieve specific goals. It is an integral part of management. A district health officer is both a manager and leader whose main role is to achieve the goals and targets of the primary health care plan. He or she may be concerned with such questions as: How can I get the job done? Which is the best way of doing that? What style of leadership should I adopt, and how can I build commitment to primary health care among the members of my team? When should I listen and when should I give orders? Will I lose the respect of my subordinates if I become friendly with them?

Role and responsibilities of the district health officer

The district health officer may have the following managerial functions:

Function	*Requirements and responsibilities*
● Formulation of district health policy	A clear understanding of national policies, priorities, and constraints, as well as district health needs and expectations. Interpretation and translation of national objectives into district objectives, targets, and plans. Preparation of budgets as part of overall district health plans. Revision of objectives, targets, and plans as necessary.
● Control of resources	Ensuring that there are good management systems in the district hospital and other health units.
● Managerial leadership	Ensuring that management structures clearly define responsibilities and accountability. Ensuring that decisions can be taken as quickly as possible. Providing managerial leadership and ensuring proper motivation of staff. Ensuring that there is effective communication among health workers. Ensuring that health workers in the district are adequately supervised and trained. Ensuring the proper planning and evaluation of health programmes.
● Establishing good relations with other sectors and communities	Developing and maintaining an effective working relationship with other sectors and communities, nongovernmental organizations, local councils, and industry. Ensuring that the needs and problems of the district are fully aired in both local and national bodies.

Delegation, supervision, and incentives

Delegation

Delegation has been defined as "investing subordinates with authority to perform the manager's job on the manager's behalf".

The starting-point in the delegation process is to examine the district health officer's own job description. Some of the jobs that have to be done can be assigned to a subordinate. Delegation can be encouraged by including a specific mention of the function in the job description of the district health officer, e.g., assignment of work to others.

Supervision

Though the supportive supervision of all health personnel is recognized as an essential factor in good management, it is often both infrequent and poor, taking the form of an "inspection" rather than a two-way learning process. An effort should be made to establish a supervisory system rather than merely organizing visits, which are only a cog in such a system. One of the main functions of supervision is to maintain and improve the quality of health care.

Supervision requires frequent (e.g. monthly) visits to all health facilities in the district. Each visit will provide information that can be used not only to allocate resources effectively, but to improve primary health care management.

On-site visits can also serve to maintain or increase staff motivation. Information to be collected should include answers to the following questions:

- What population is served?

- What is the staffing pattern?

- What services are currently provided?

- What is the present coverage by various programmes?

- Are outreach activities currently provided?

- Are the logistics — supplies and equipment — adequate?

- How are the equipment and facilities maintained?

- How is the work organized?

- What problems hamper the current operation of the facility? How are the staff tackling these problems?

- What suggestions do the staff have on how activities might be improved?

With the immense variety of resources and types of terrain involved, great flexibility, innovation, and imagination are needed (especially as regards logistics) in establishing subsystems for supervision at district and subdistrict level. The whole effort should be based, at least initially, on the realities of the local situation and the resources available. Alternative ways of providing supportive supervision need to be explored. For example, in many countries, health centres are supposed to supervise subcentres and community health workers. The distances involved are sometimes more than 100 km, and the absence of reliable means of transport makes reasonable supervision impossible. In such circumstances, should supportive supervision be the responsibility of the district team? If so, vehicles need to be provided at district level. Or should the use of bicycles and other cheaper means of transport be encouraged? Some countries tackle the problem by holding supervisory meetings every month, on the day when the community health workers come to the health centre to collect drugs and discuss their problems. Similarly, the responsible officers of health centres meet once a month at the district hospital.

It goes without saying that, for effective supervision, it is important to set a good personal example. This rule, however, is not always observed — witness the case of a district health manager who was furious with his community health workers for demanding remuneration, though it was well known in the district that, in addition to his relatively high salary, he was raking in considerable amounts of money from an illegal private practice.

Incentives

Sometimes training, redefinition of tasks, and supervision will not be enough by themselves to motivate health workers adequately. It is necessary to improve both the status and financial rewards of all staff, particularly those working in rural areas. It is unrealistic to expect good performances under difficult conditions from workers who are poorly rewarded. A whole range of incentives are used in different countries, for example, an annual prize for the best district, health centre, doctor, nurse, etc; a certificate from the head of state for the best worker; scholarships and fellowships; salary increases for specific achievements; subsidized housing to encourage residence in rural areas; and various awards for rural work, such as degrees or salary increments. The aim of such incentives should be to encourage a wide range of approaches to the task of meeting the health needs of the population. Too often the main problem is not poor organization, inadequate management, or lack of skills, but low morale.

Supplies, logistics, and maintenance

Adequate support for primary health care demands efficient handling of drugs and supplies, including their procurement, distribution, and transport, as well as the maintenance of buildings and equipment and, sometimes, minor construction work. The procurement of vaccines, medicines and supplies frequently poses problems. A decision is needed as to which items should be purchased regularly. Are the current organizational systems for distribution satisfactory? Does the district health organization have enough control over them? Does the district operate an essential drugs and equipment list? Are storage facilities, including cold-chain facilities, available,

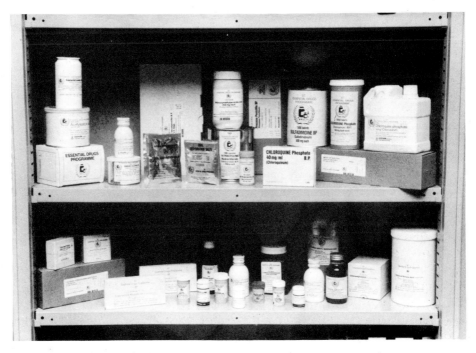

Essential drugs are those that meet the health care needs of the majority of the population.
Photo WHO/J. Germain (19333)

adequate and functioning? Are there adequate means of transport? Are they properly used? Are transport facilities and equipment adequately maintained? Where there is a shortage of motorized transport, what alternatives, such as bicycles, horses, etc., are available? These are but some of the issues that the district health team has to address in the area of logistics.

To improve logistics, it is useful to start by reviewing the most important functions such as:

- planning and budgeting
- receiving and inspecting
- storage and warehousing
- inventory control
- supply
- distribution and transport
- maintenance and repair
- communications
- records and reporting.

The steps required to fulfil these functions must be determined, and it must then be asked whether each of them can in fact be carried out. For example, it is worth asking:

- Is there a specified supply period?
- Are stock records up-to-date?
- Is the quantity of items used during the supply period known?
- What is the wastage rate for major items?
- Are there adequate stocks of requisition forms?
- Are there adequate staff to make requisitions and check paperwork?
- Have re-order levels for major stock items been established?
- Are reserve stocks maintained?

Recording systems and checklists must be devised, so that logistic activities can be regularly maintained and controlled. Fig. 9 provides an example of a stock record card that might be used for inventory control.

Date	Document number	Issued to/ rec'd from	Received	Issued	Balance	Initials	Date	Document number	Issued to/ rec'd from	Received	Issued	Balance	Initials

STOCK RECORD CARD
MINISTRY OF HEALTH
Department of Medical Supply

Description:_____
Stock no:_____
Unit of issue:_____
Bin location:_____
Alternatives:_____

Estimated monthly
consumption:_____

Reorder level:_____
Order quantity:_____
Maximum level:_____
Review period:_____
Safety stock:_____

Fig. 9. Sample stock record card

Financial management

The district health team has overall responsibility for the preparation and management of the budget. The hallmark of an experienced district health officer is the ability to use resources efficiently. The cost of various alternatives needs to be worked out and taken into account when making decisions. This calls for information on unit costs, including those for hospital beds and outpatient attendance.

There are three main financial considerations at district level: the ways in which resources are allocated and controlled by officials at more central levels; the allocation of resources within the district; and the mobilization and use of local financial resources for primary health care. District-level staff need to ensure that the collection and expenditure of locally mobilized resources are accounted for. Budgets allocated at higher levels will vary in the degree of flexibility with which they can be used at the district and local levels. Greater flexibility is needed for the adequate support of local needs than for the execution of a programme of predetermined services.

Relevant questions include the following: Can revenue and resources be raised locally and, if so, what is the best way of managing them? How far can budgetary allocations be adjusted to local circumstances? How do the allocations compare with actual expenditure? Can expenditure be transferred between budgetary allocations?

There must be budgetary control. In managing plans and programmes, it is necessary to keep track of expenditure. When money is voted for projects, it will usually be divided among various lines of expenditure. Knowing

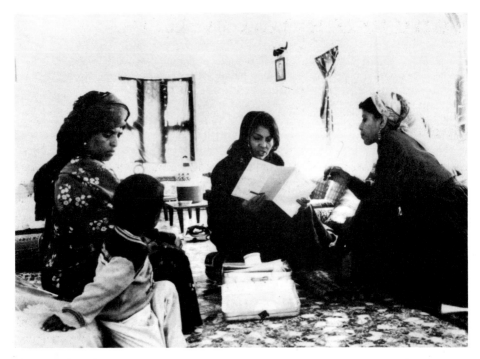

Health workers are gradually learning to use fewer drugs in a more rational way. *Photo WHO/M. Jacot (19643)*

whether the money has been spent on time is one way of assessing how well the plan or programme is progressing. If there has been overspending or underspending under a particular line, the reasons must be worked out at a management meeting.

CHAPTER 8

Monitoring and control

Monitoring

Monitoring is the process of measuring, coordinating, collecting, processing, and communicating information of assistance to management and decision-making. It is an essential part of the implementation phase of a programme, since it provides feedback. Its purpose is to identify immediate problems or deviations from the established plan and find quick practical solutions. Monitoring is based on a comparison between established norms or standards and actual performance.

The sources of information used in monitoring health activities include monthly, quarterly, and annual reports from health centres and hospitals, data on notifiable diseases, and special surveys. The format of the reports will vary according to the nature of the activities being monitored. Table 7 shows data that might be included in a quarterly report from a health centre. The inclusion of information on the achievement of goals (for example, reductions in case-fatality rates and maternal mortality) may be of some help in assessing the quality of care.

Good information systems are required for effective monitoring. Many forms and registers are kept at local health units, but often these are not used or analysed. Data are usually collected and passed on to higher echelons. These too are rarely, if ever, analysed. The data frequently consist of requests from individual, uncoordinated, vertical programmes, each with its own reporting format; unfortunately, this is seldom appropriate for planning at district level. Simple procedures for collecting information to be used at the local level and to provide feedback to other levels need to be devised. To this end, decisions must be made about the forms and registers to be kept at the various units in the district. It must be emphasized that the problem is not a shortage of data — there is often too much—but the fact that little useful information can be gleaned from them.

Sources of information

Major sources of information include: routine reporting; recording of tracer diseases; sentinel sites; supervisory visits, and community diagnosis.

Table 7. Suggested layout for a health centre's quarterly report

(i)	Population covered . . . . . . Percentage of women of reproductive age			
(ii)	Births registered . . . . .expected			
(iii)	Deaths			
(iv)	Children under 5 who are underweight			
(v)	Family planning users			
(vi)	Antenatal visits . . . . Antenatal visits per mother . . . . Percentage of antenatal visits during first 6 months of pregnancy			

(vii) Immunization

BCG	. . . .	% of those eligible	. . . .
DPT-I	. . . .		. . . .
-II	. . . .		. . . .
Polio-I	. . . .		. . . .
-II	. . . .		. . . .
Measles	. . . .		. . . .
Tetanus toxoid	. . . .		. . . .

(viii)	Outpatient attendances	. . . .	
(ix)	No. of inpatients	. . . .	

Normal recording and reporting

Data routinely kept by health workers on attendance at health facilities come under this heading. In addition, there are the data on families and the population recorded by some facilities. Family cards or folders are used to keep salient information, including the sex and date of birth of each family member. Health events are recorded on a separate page. Many peripheral health facilities, which provide the first contact with families, also keep maps, indicating (*a*) catchment area, population, and population distribution; and (*b*) homes, schools, and streets.

Tracer diseases

Detailed surveillance and recording of selected diseases may be more useful than attempting to note everything down. In this case, only the tracer diseases are recorded in detail, others being noted only in a general way. Some of the factors to be taken into consideration in the selection of tracer diseases or problems are:

- Does the disease or problem occur with sufficient frequency to allow reasonable numbers of cases to be detected?

- Can the harm from the disease or problem be significantly reduced by an appropriate intervention?

- Is successful intervention conditional on activities that can be modified?

Measles is an example of a possible tracer disease in many developing countries. Immunization is an effective preventive measure. But successful measles immunization depends on the viability of the vaccine, which is a sensitive indicator of the efficiency of the health system logistics in the district and country and the quality of the cold chain. The coverage will also depend on community awareness and mobilization of resources. Finally, the severity of measles in a community is a good indication of the nutritional status of its children.

Another example is anaemia, the incidence of which gives some idea of the effectiveness of malaria control and environmental sanitation programmes. Similarly, the incidence of acute diarrhoea is a useful indicator of progress in environmental sanitation and diarrhoeal disease control. Table 8 shows conditions that have been used as tracers by some countries.

Sentinel sites

As well as endeavouring to improve reporting throughout the district, it may be useful to select a few representative urban and rural facilities whose reports are particularly reliable and can be used as indicators of what is happening in the district. Since sentinel sites are like watchmen, giving a warning of impending problems, every attempt should be made to include facilities suspected of having difficulties in implementing the programme, so that the worst possible situations may be monitored. Governmental and nongovernmental facilities should be involved where they serve an appreciable proportion of the population. Sentinel sites should be chosen to

Table 8. Tracer conditions applicable to different age groups (males and females)

Tracer condition

Age group (years)	measles	middle ear infection	malaria	hearing loss	vision defect	iron deficiency anaemia	hyper-tension	urinary tract infection	cervical cancer
Females									
Under 5	+	+	+			+			
5–24		+	+	+	+				
25–64						+	+	+	+
65 & over						+	+	+	+
Males									
Under 5	+	+	+			+			
5–24		+	+	+	+				
25–64						+	+		
65 & over						+	+	+	

represent certain geographical areas, and on the basis of the willingness of the personnel to participate and the existence of a reasonably good and usable recording system.

Supervisory visits

Supervisory visits provide an opportunity for assessment of facilities and of patient satisfaction. Scoring systems can be used, points being awarded for cleanliness of premises, state of the refrigerator, community programmes, knowledge of patients, etc.

Community diagnosis

Data kept by community health workers, supplemented by surveys when necessary, provide useful information on community health.

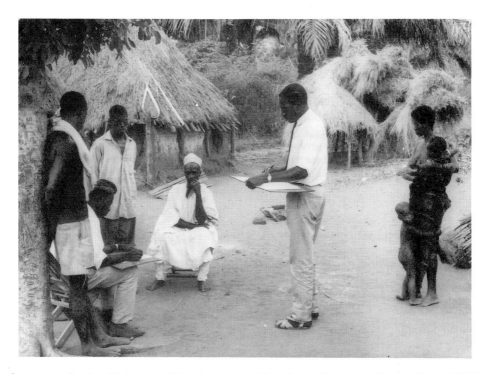

A community health worker interviewing families in a Nigerian village. *Photo WHO/ D. Henrioud (12526)*

Estimates

The prevalence of many endemic diseases can be assessed on the basis of estimates from average national rates or published review data.

Information should be presented in the form of graphs, bar charts, or maps, where this is useful. For example, graphs showing the seasonal variation in the number of deaths may indicate impending outbreaks of disease. Similarly, a graph indicating the percentage of eligible children vaccinated will show whether real progress is being made in the immunization programme. Comparisons between the data on the health situation and the availability of health care for different geographical areas and population groups will make it possible to assess how far the distribution of health care is equitable.

Control

Control is the managerial function that keeps the plan or programme within tolerable limits relative to its targets. Essentially, control involves the following activities:

- selecting indicators and milestones that reflect actual performance

- gathering and analysing information on the performance of projects measured against plans, indicators, and timetables

- establishing the procedures for taking corrective action if excessive deviations from the plan occur.

It is important to identify what is controllable in a plan or programme. This depends on the nature and authority of the management team and the range of control tools and techniques considered. However, the chief items to be controlled include:

- organization of personnel

- assignment of functions and responsibilities

- financial performance in terms of allocation and expenditure

- project assets, facilities, machinery, equipment, and any capital items at the project's disposal (proper use, maintenance, repair, security, etc.)

- correspondence (which must be maintained, monitored, and properly adapted to project needs and performance)

● reports, logistics, and services, e.g., immunization.

The visual presentation of data and plans, using, for example, Gantt charts and graphs, should be encouraged. The Gantt chart (Table 9) is one of the simplest, yet probably the most useful, of the well-known management control devices. It is a simple horizontal bar chart showing the beginning and end points of specific activities or tasks that are needed to carry out a programme or project. It shows at a glance the chronological relationship of activities—where they overlap or are in parallel with one another, when they start and finish.

Table 9. Use of Gantt chart for conducting a survey

Activity	Responsible officer	Jan	Feb	Mar	Apr	May	Jun
Briefing of district leaders	ET	X...................... X					
Briefing of villagers	HK				X..............................X		
Design of survey	DS			X..................X			
Selection and training of staff	JM			X..................X			
Conduct of survey	AH					X..................X	
Analysis of report	AG						X...
Provision of transport and logistic support	AI	X...X					

CHAPTER 9

Evaluation and learning by doing

Evaluation

Evaluation of the implementation of a district primary health care plan or programme is a more comprehensive form of assessment than regular monitoring. Monitoring leads to changes in plans of action; evaluation may lead to wholesale reformulation of priorities and plans. Evaluation is a systematic way of learning from experience and using the lessons learned to improve current activities and promote better plans by the careful selection of alternatives for future action. This involves analysis of the different phases of a programme, its relevance, formulation, efficiency and effectiveness, and the extent of its acceptance by all parties involved. It renders possible the reallocation of priorities and resources on the basis of changing health needs.

Evaluation may not necessarily cover all aspects of primary health care, but should include the following criteria: effectiveness, equity, efficiency, and impact:

- *Effectiveness* is an expression of the degree of attainment of the predetermined objectives and targets of a programme, institution, or activity seeking to reduce a health problem or improve an unsatisfactory health situation. This factor depends on whether the various activities and measures undertaken work (efficacy) and the degree to which they are accepted by those for whom they are intended.

- *Equity* considers the coverage of population groups and geographical areas, distribution of resources and facilities, and effectiveness of services in different areas. Equity in the distribution of health care depends on the extent to which different geographical areas and population groups, according to age, sex, or wealth, have access to essential services.

- *Efficiency* is an expression of the relationship between the results obtained from a health programme or activity and the efforts expended in terms of human, financial, and other resources, health processes, technology, and time. The reason for assessing efficiency is to improve implementation and gain a better idea of the progress made.

● *Impact* is an expression of the overall effect of a programme, service, or institution on health and related aspects of socioeconomic development. The assessment of impact thus aims at identifying any necessary change in the direction of health programmes, so as to replan primary health care accordingly and increase its contribution to health and overall socioeconomic development.

The description of these components of evaluation would be incomplete without some reference to the question of frequency. While the evaluation may be a continuing process, the results have to be summarized and reported on at given times or at specified intervals. Experience throughout the world shows that health systems tend to be rigid, resisting change and often continuing to operate in the same way year after year. Unless the functioning of the system is reviewed periodically, there is a danger that it will become fossilized or change only in times of financial crisis. It may be easier to summarize progress and efficiency, say, once a year, than to assess effectiveness, for which a longer interval may be required, since significant long-term changes in the health situation will have to be identified. An even longer period is likely to be needed before impact can be assessed—perhaps five years or more from the inception of a programme.

The evaluation process

The evaluation process begins with an appraisal of the objectives of the programme and setting of standards. Evaluation can be carried out on each of the components of the district planning cycle.

As regards the first component of the cycle—national policies and guidance—it is important to evaluate the extent to which district plans and activities conform to national policies. How effective is the national planning process as seen in the districts? Is decentralization adequate? Is effective guidance provided on options for organizing and financing health care? How effective and efficient is support from the national level with regard to planning services, joint action, and management?

Concerning the next three components—analysis of the present situation, appraisal of district priorities, and setting objectives and targets—it is important to know, among other things, how efficiently these processes have been carried out. Has optimal information been obtained? Information is costly to collect and an excessive amount may overwhelm the system, thus obscuring important considerations. Were the costs of alternatives taken into account?

In district action programmes, indicators for evaluation include the efficient utilization of health care, the equitable distribution of such care, and the technical efficiency of health services. Overutilization is evidenced by unnecessarily high figures for per capita consumption of drugs, hospital admissions, performance of certain surgical procedures, and professional consultations per year. Underutilization occurs either because the services are unwanted and thus bypassed, or because the supply exceeds the demand.

Table 10 provides further examples of criteria for evaluation. Levels of performance in meeting these criteria could be classed as: (1) standards consistently met; (2) standards often met; (3) standards sometimes met; (4) standards occasionally met; and (5) standards not met.

The best district

A number of countries regularly award prizes to the best district and/or district health officer and other health workers. This appears to be an excellent way of improving the functioning of district health systems, especially if the selection of winners is done in public, using explicit criteria. The criteria and standards given in Table 10, modified as necessary, might be useful in this exercise. Both qualitative and quantitative indicators are used, and the decision will depend on which features of district health systems are to be emphasized in the assessment.

Table 10. Standards for the evaluation of a district health system

1. *Plan of action.* There should be a district plan of action with all the following features:

- It is based on a systematic assessment of the existing situation.
- The process of development allowed for wide consultation.
- It is reviewed annually.
- Clear priorities and targets have been established.
- Costs have been estimated.
- It provides the following:
  - curative services, including quality control
  - maternal and child health services, including immunization and family planning
  - health promotion services, services for the prevention and control of communicable and noncommunicable diseases
  - environmental and occupational health services
  - outreach programmes.

Table 10 (contd.)

2. *Joint action.* There should be:

- a multisectoral district advisory committee or a subcommittee of the district develop- ment committee, which meets regularly and keeps minutes of decisions
- multisectoral village development committees where health matters are discussed
- cooperation with nongovernmental organizations and with religious and political organizations
- cooperation with traditional birth attendants
- cooperation with other traditional practitioners
- cooperation with communities in the selection of community health workers.

3. *Improved management.* There should be:

- a chart of the organizational structure that is easily available
- a staffing table
- a list of essential equipment and drugs for all units
- an effort to attain at least national norms for staffing levels
- job descriptions for all staff categories
- regular meetings of the district management team, with minutes available
- refresher courses for all staff at least once every three years
- a staff incentive programme
- a chronological record of expenditure
- availability of drugs and other essential supplies throughout the year
- availability of essential means of transport.

4. *Monitoring.* There should be:

- district monthly reports (available by the middle of the subsequent month)
- reports by all health units (available by the middle of the subsequent month)
- visual presentation of information.

5. *Evaluation and learning by doing.* There should be:

- an evaluation committee to assess progress and programme quality
- established methods of assessment and standards
- quarterly meetings of the committee
- follow-up of the committee's findings
- systematic action to find solutions to difficulties encountered in the district.

6. *Impact.* This is reflected in:

- improved organization and management of district health systems (1–5 above)
- increased coverage with essential care.

Findings could be recorded as follows:

- percentage of population within 5 km of a health facility
- percentage of female population who are literate

Table 10 (contd.)

- percentage of population with clean water in compound or within 15 minutes' walk
- percentage of houses (families) with latrines
- percentage of mothers receiving care during first three months of pregnancy
- percentage of mothers attended at childbirth by trained health worker
- percentage of children fully immunized
- percentage of eligible couples who are practising family planning
- decrease in percentage of newborns with weight less than 2500 g
- percentage decrease in morbidity and mortality from major endemic diseases
- percentage decrease in infant mortality rate
- percentage decrease in maternal mortality
- decrease in percentage of inequities in health and health care between geographical areas and population groups.

Learning by doing

The purpose of evaluation, as described above, is to determine the extent to which programmes and services are actually working and achieving operational targets and results in terms of health. Often, however, the likely effects of new programmes and methods of delivering care are not at all clear. Under these circumstances, some research may be needed to determine the most appropriate way forward. For example, to what extent should village health workers be provided with drugs to dispense to the local population? The answer to this question might be obtained by setting up a trial in which different ranges of drugs are given to groups of village health workers, and then assessing how appropriately they prescribe them and how well the patients comply with their instructions. To help evaluation, studies of this nature can be carried out on an *ad hoc* basis in preselected areas.

An unfortunate tendency in health care is for outside "experts" to claim that the appropriate solutions are known and that the challenge is one of implementation. If, for example, the government is not providing sufficient funds for primary health care, this is said to be due to lack of political will. Training is the usual answer to poor performance by community health workers at health centres or hospitals. A sense of humility is needed, together with a willingness to acknowledge that a gap between expert opinion and people's traditional wisdom is a problem.

Operational research

Operational research often has wide relevance and applicability and, if designed and carried out adequately, may be applicable to a number of districts. Indeed, since such research is time-consuming, it is imperative that districts should learn from studies carried out elsewhere. In some countries it may be useful to have selected areas or districts which, together with supporting institutions and experts at the national level, could undertake practical research. In fact, a number of such districts already exist in different parts of the world. These are not pilot districts in the usual sense.

It is essential that the provision of technical cooperation to selected areas or districts, whether by national institutions or from external sources, should be channelled in such a way that there is no risk of their becoming so different from other areas that the lessons learnt will be inapplicable to the rest of the country. The research should be continued for a specific period of time, so that if a new initiative is shown to be unsuccessful, it can be abandoned and not implemented elsewhere. New initiatives often become self-fulfilling and are adopted widely without any real evaluation of the benefit to the population.

Some of the innovations to be introduced in the selected districts—for example, comprehensive maternal and child health clinics or the deployment of community health workers—may already have been attempted with varying degrees of success in other districts. But such innovations are rarely, if ever, subjected to rigorous experimental assessment. It is this essential element, the equivalent of the randomized clinical trial of medical procedures, which is being stressed here. The precise forms of innovation to be tried will vary from time to time; they should all be monitored and documented, and the information obtained made available to other districts. Without this approach, change will be based only on intuition and learning will be difficult.

The following are examples of areas in which studies may be required:

- Is it possible to develop resource allocation methods that promote a better use of resources in relation to population needs? Among other things, it is important to know the present pattern of expenditure—governmental, private, nongovernmental, etc.—as well as the overall financial resources of the health sector in the district.

- How can a districtwide health information system be developed which could help to define the problems of the population and support decision-making at all levels of the health services, including hospitals?

This question calls for detailed studies of the strengths and weaknesses of the present system.

- How can priority-setting be related more closely to the impact of various interventions?

- How can the first-referral hospital become more fully linked with other facilities in the district health system?

- What would be a more efficient system of health care delivery?

- What types of health unit should be in the system? Should there be health centres, subcentres, and dispensaries, or health centres only?

- What is the optimum staffing pattern?

- How should maternal and child health and the control of malaria, tuberculosis, and leprosy be integrated with primary health care?

- How can the organization of services within units, e.g., the flow of patients, be improved?

- Are services reaching those in need? Who uses them and why?

- How can services keep up with ever-changing patterns of ill-health?

- How can supervision be improved?

Such studies should facilitate monitoring and evaluation and permit recommendations for the strengthening of district services to be made on the basis of sound evidence that they are worth while. Districts can then adopt new strategies that are known to work, to improve primary health care.

References

1. *Glossary of terms used in the "Health for All" Series No. 1–8.* Geneva, World Health Organization, 1984 ("Health for All" Series, No. 9).
2. *Eighth General Programme of Work covering the period 1990–1995.* Geneva, World Health Organization, 1987 ("Health for All" Series, No. 10).
3. TABIBZADEH, I. ET AL. *Spotlight on the cities: improving urban health in developing countries.* Geneva, World Health Organization, 1989.
4. *Broad programming as a part of the managerial process for national health development. Guiding principles.* Unpublished WHO document MPNHD/81.3. Available on request from Planning, Coordination and Cooperation, World Health Organization, 1211 Geneva 27, Switzerland.
5. HELANDER, E. ET AL. *Training in the community for people with disabilities.* Geneva, World Health Organization, 1989.
6. BRÈS, P. *Public health action in emergencies caused by epidemics.* Geneva, World Health Organization, 1986.
7. FRANCEYS, R. ET AL. *A guide to the development of on-site sanitation.* Geneva, World Health Organization, in preparation.
8. SUESS, M. J. *Solid waste management. Selected topics.* Copenhagen, WHO Regional Office for Europe, 1985.
9. *Health principles of housing.* Geneva, World Health Organization, 1989.
10. *Drug dependence and alcohol-related problems. A manual for community health workers with guidelines for trainers.* Geneva, World Health Organization, 1986.
11. *The introduction of a mental health component into primary health care.* Geneva, World Health Organization, 1990.
12. ROEMER, M. I. & MONTOYA-AGUILAR, C. *Quality assessment and assurance in primary health care.* Geneva, World Health Organization, 1988 (WHO Offset Publication, No. 105).